THE SURGICAL NEONATE

THE SURGICAL NEONATE

EVALUATION AND CARE

HOWARD C. FILSTON, M.D.

Associate Professor of Pediatric Surgery and Pediatrics
Chief of Pediatric Surgical Service
Duke University Medical Center
Durham, North Carolina

ROBERT IZANT, JR., M.D.

Professor of Pediatric Surgery
Chief of Pediatric Surgery
Case Western Reserve University
School of Medicine
Cleveland, Ohio

To William Schuchardt – a fine person and surgical resident – Robert J Izant Jr June 1978

ACC

APPLETON-CENTURY-CROFTS / New York

78 79 80 81 82 / 10 9 8 7 6 5 4 3 2 1

Prentice-Hall International, Inc., London
Prentice-Hall of Australia, Pty. Ltd., Sydney
Prentice-Hall of India Private Limited, New Delhi
Prentice-Hall of Japan, Inc., Tokyo
Prentice-Hall of Southeast Asia (Pte.) Ltd., Singapore
Whitehall Books, Ltd., Wellington, New Zealand

Library of Congress Cataloging in Publication Data

Filston, Howard C
The surgical neonate.

Includes index.
1. Infants (Newborn)—Surgery. I. Izant, Robert J. joint author. II. Title. [DNLM: 1. Infant, Newborn, Diseases—Surgery. 2. Postoperative care—In infancy and childhood. 3. Preoperative care—In infancy and childhood. 4. Surgery—In infancy and childhood. WO925 D489s]
RD137.5.F54 617'.98 77–26020

Text design: Millicent Fairhurst
Cover design: B. Andrew Mudryk

PRINTED IN THE UNITED STATES OF AMERICA

0-8385-8716-X

To Nancy Lee and Virginia

CONTENTS

ACKNOWLEDGMENTS

How little of a work such as this is one's own! Beyond the many theories and procedures that can be specifically referenced are the even more important ideas and techniques that one's many teachers and colleagues have shared so freely over the years. As the principal author, I am usurping the privilege of writing these acknowledgments, so that I can express my gratitude to my long-time teacher, colleague, associate, and coauthor, Robert James Izant, Jr., for the standards of excellence that he has taught me and the many years of encouragement and support that he has given me.

This book had its infancy as a small handout at the Children's Hospital of Philadelphia. Much that is good in it is but a compendium of the teachings of C. Everett Koop, Harry Bishop, Dale Johnson, Patricia Bornes, and Jack Downes.

I have had the good fortune in my career to be associated with outstanding neonatologists from whom I have learned much about the care of tiny infants. These include Marshall Klaus and Avroy Fanaroff at Rainbow Babies' and Children's Hospital and George Brumley, Lillian Blackmon, and Jane Brazy at Duke University. Robert Crumrine, chief of pediatric anesthesia at Case Western Reserve University, provided the bridge between neonatology and safe anesthesia and respiratory care.

In many ways this book owes its inception to William Drucker's challenge to learn something about vascular volume deficiency and tissue perfusion, for it stems from an attempt to apply the rapidly evolving knowledge of shock mechanisms and volume maintenance to infants.

Many house officers have used the various unpublished manuals that preceded this book, and their comments and criticisms have been helpful. However, only Bruce Smith at Duke University really tore it apart paragraph by paragraph as I had hoped someone would do. Then he kindly took the time and great effort to help me put it back together again!

I am thankful for the support of William D. Holden, C. Everett Koop, and David C. Sabiston, Jr., outstanding leaders of American surgery, who took the time to review this work and encouraged me to see it through to completion. The Audiovisual Department at Duke Medical Center and particularly Charles Lewis, Jr., were most helpful in preparing the illustrations. Finally, my two secretaries, Jane Van Bergen in Cleveland, who typed the manuscript through so many revisions, and Barbara Shaw in Durham, who took on a new boss, a new specialty, and the final expansion and revision of a new book all at the same time, made the book possible by their patience and excellent work. My thanks go also to the publisher, Appleton-Century-Crofts and in particular to Robert E. McGrath and Barbara A. Bullied for publishing the book as we wanted it to be.

HCF

PREFACE

Pediatric surgery is a young specialty with few fully trained surgeons and even fewer training programs. Even in most major teaching centers in this country the pediatric surgery service is staffed primarily by residents and interns from general surgery and pediatrics who rotate through for brief periods with little prior knowledge of the field. Available time does not permit them to read extensively in the standard textbooks in the field, and the available handbooks try to be too all inclusive and therefore are lacking in needed pragmatic details.

We have endeavored to present, not a broad outline of the whole field of pediatric surgery, but rather a thorough introduction to the management of the surgical newborn in the hope that it will rapidly orient the house officer, student, or physician who occasionally must deal with newborn surgical anomalies, to the important factors in diagnosis and management. Through this educational effort we would hope for improved care and reduced mortality for the neonate and young infant.

The evolution of pediatric surgery as a specialty field has been a history of increasing involvement with the newborn. The pediatric surgeon has a special contribution to make because he is familiar with the characteristics of the multitude of unusual abnormalities that are surgically correctable and is interested in and knowledgeable about the unique physiologic requirements for homeostasis in the newborn period. The successful correction of a major congenital defect is not merely a feat of operative technique. Rather, it is the summation of an intensive team effort on the part of knowledgeable specialists in neonatology, pediatric anesthesia, pediatric surgery, and appropriate consulting specialties. Each contributes his own expertise while having sufficient knowledge of the overall physiologic problems to recognize the importance of the others' contributions.

Since the vast majority of newborns are normal at birth, the rare surgical problems that characterize the neonatal period can create confusion, doubt, and inappropriate action by the attending physicians. How to anticipate, recognize, and evaluate a neonatal surgical problem, expedite preoperative preparation, and intelligently manage postoperative care are the subjects of this book.

The book is divided into three major sections. The first two sections are intended as a source of general knowledge. Section I details the overall management of the newborn infant before, during, and after surgery. It includes chapters on fluid and electrolytes, evaluation and general care, monitoring, and airway management. In Section II, the most frequent presenting symptom complexes are discussed from the standpoint of differential diagnosis and urgency of treatment. Section III contains important additional material on numerous congenital anomalies, but it is intended primarily to be a ready reference source for planning initial management of infants whose diagnosis is known or suspected. Some of the material presented in Section II is therefore repeated in Section III to save hunting for it when a quick reference source is required.

The photo at left shows Erik. Born weighing 1900 g, he was found to have esophageal atresia and distal tracheoesophageal fistula. Severe aspiration pneumonia prevented early corrective surgery, and his esophagus was eventually repaired in three stages. Recrudescence of pneumonia and severe sepsis required tracheostomy and mechanical ventilation for three and a half months, during which time he sustained twelve cardiac arrests requiring resuscitation. Central total parenteral nutrition maintained his nitrogen balance and provided needed nutrition for growth for most of that time. Finally discharged from the hospital at five months of age, he required almost three years of frequent dilations before his esophagus functioned entirely normally. At four years of age, he is a normal, healthy, happy fully functioning child. Erik is what this book is all about.

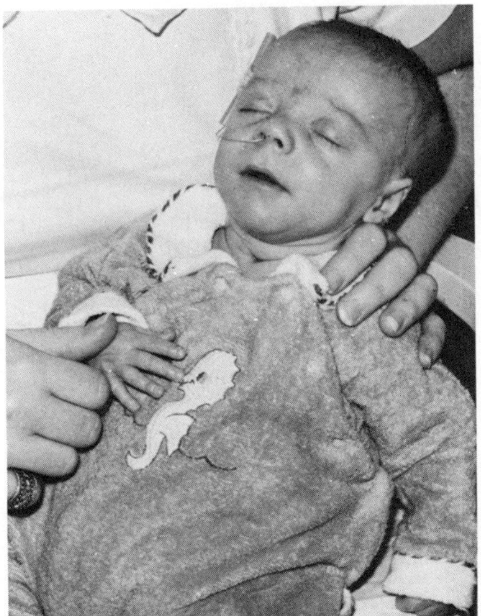

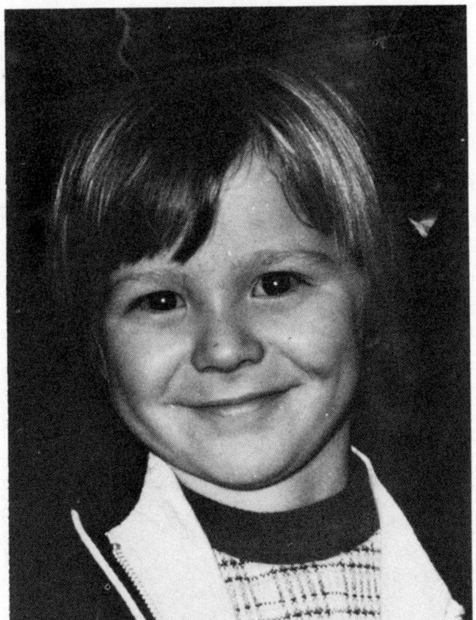

THE SURGICAL NEONATE

SECTION 1

GENERAL MANAGEMENT OF THE NEONATE

Before embarking on a presentation of the various symptom complexes that represent surgical lesions in the neonate, some discussion of the management of the physiologic derangements of surgical illnesses is essential. The physician caring for a neonate with a surgically treatable illness, whether he is a pediatrician or surgeon, must adhere to those principles of temperature control, fluid and electrolyte maintenance, respiratory evaluation and support, acid/base control, and thorough investigation of related pathophysiologic entities that are required to insure homeostasis in the face of added burdens of surgical disease, anesthesia, and operative trauma.

The emphasis in Section I is on the important facets of vascular volume restoration in the preoperative and postoperative periods, together with some discussion of the principles of total intravenous alimentation (total parenteral nutrition), a significant new technique that has proved to be valuable not only to the patient with a surgical lesion, but to many newborns and young infants with chronic metabolic and biochemical derangements. For these infants, a period of improved nutrition and gastrointestinal rest may be the deciding factor for improvement. The final chapters in Section I discuss the overall management of the newborn, modern monitoring techniques, and management of the neonatal airway.

CHAPTER 1

PARENTERAL FLUID AND ELECTROLYTE MANAGEMENT

INTRODUCTION TO PEDIATRIC FLUID AND ELECTROLYTE MANAGEMENT

The past 15 years have seen vast changes in the management of fluids and electrolytes in surgical patients. In the mid-1950s, after metabolic experiments in Boston seemed to show an inappropriate sodium and water retention after surgery, sodium and water restriction became the guiding principles of postoperative management.[1] With extensive investigations into shock in the early 1960s came appreciation of the hypovolemic tendencies of the postsurgical patient.[2–4] Finally, it was demonstrated that the antidiuretic hormone could be "shut off" if adequate extracellular fluid (ECF) replacement fluids were given.[5–8] More recently, evaluations of third-space fluid shifts during and after surgery and anesthesia have led to inappropriate emphasis on overexpansion of the extracellular fluid volume with electrolyte solutions.[9]

Pediatric surgical fluid and electrolyte management, at least as discussed in the literature and texts, has tended to lag behind advances in adult management. This has resulted from an overemphasis of the differences between infant and adult kidneys in the handling of fluid loads and salt.[10–12] Although certain known differences in the premature infant's physiology demand careful modification of any general program of fluid management, we believe that the premature newborn as well as the infant and older child can be managed by a well thought out general program seeking optimal replacement of vascular volume with consequent good tissue perfusion and corresponding optimal renal function and urine output.[13–16] It is to this end that the following management program is directed.

DAILY FLUID AND ELECTROLYTE REQUIREMENTS IN PEDIATRIC SURGICAL PATIENTS BY CATEGORY

MAINTENANCE

Water and Calories

This volume is based on requirements for replacement of insensible loss from skin and lungs and *obligatory* urine needed to clear metabolic wastes, particularly urea. Insensible loss probably averages about 40 to 50 ml/kg per day.[17] Adequate urine for clearing wastes without extreme concentration demands on the kidney equals about 40 ml/kg per day.[17] Guidelines have been worked out in metabolic balance studies for caloric and fluid needs per square meter body surface area per day. The slope of a line graph defining calories per square meter per day is equal to (100 − 3× age in years) (weight in kilograms). This formula approximates the maintenance fluid requirements but provides far fewer than normal calories, if given in standard solutions (eg 5 percent dextrose/one-fifth normal saline).

FORMULA: DAILY MAINTENANCE WATER

(100 ml − 3× age in years)(weight in kilograms)[17]

We consider 1500 ml a good restrictive level for maintenance in the adult. Therefore, when the formula calculations reach above 1500 ml, this level is held to.

EXCEPTIONS TO MAINTENANCE FORMULA

1. Neonates (for 48 hours postoperatively): 1 to 2 days of age, 65 ml/kg per 24 hours; 2 to 7 days of age, 85 ml/kg per 24 hours. Note: This reduction presupposes that sizable volumes of electrolyte solutions are being given for internal fluid shifts and that urine output is being closely monitored.
2. Diabetes insipidus: More free water is usually needed.
3. Increased perspiration or prolonged high fever: More water and maintenance electrolytes must be given.
4. Hypertonic electrolytes or hyperosmolar states: Increased free water and decreased maintenance electrolytes are needed to achieve dilution.
5. Hypotonic dehydrations: Decrease the amounts of hypotonic maintenance solutions and give maintenance volumes plus calculated re-

placement volumes in solutions containing full levels of electrolytes such as 5 percent dextrose/normal saline (D_5/NS) or 5 percent dextrose/Ringer's lactate (D_5/RL).

6. Hypotonic normovolemic: Decrease hypotonic maintenance solutions and give maintenance volumes in full-level electrolyte solutions to allow correction as free water is utilized for insensible losses.
7. Hypotonic hypervolemic (as when the postoperative patient begins to mobilize his third-space fluids on the third or fourth postoperative day): Reduce total fluid to maintenance and give as full electrolyte solutions.
8. Severe cardiac decompensation: Reduce maintenance volumes to minimal levels.
9. Hyperventilation states (eg, diabetic acidosis and burn patients being treated with mafenide acetate*): Increased volumes of free water for increased insensible loss from lung may be needed.
10. Ultrasonic mist: Drastic reductions in maintenance hypotonic solutions may be needed because of potential large-volume absorption through the bronchiolar and possibly alveolar membranes. Reduce maintenance in neonates to 50 ml/kg to begin.

NOTE

In no instance other than the above exceptions is the volume of maintenance hypotonic solution changed from that calculated by the formula. Specifically, the volumes of these hypotonic solutions, eg, D_5/0.25 NS, are not increased regardless of total fluid requirements. In most instances additional fluid requirements are the result of either specific measurable losses or third-space shifts and must be replaced with solutions containing full levels of electrolytes, if normal serum electrolyte levels are to be maintained. Unnecessary hypotonic fluids given in the presence of hypovolemia and antidiuretic hormone will be retained and shifted into the tissues along the osmotic concentration gradient. This can lead to peripheral and, more dangerously, interstitial pulmonary edema.

Sodium Chloride

The maintenance volume is 3 mEq/kg per day (up to 45 mEq). Five percent dextrose/0.25 NS has about 3.8 mEq/100 ml. Therefore, maintenance water and sodium chloride will usually be provided by the volumes of

*Sulfamylon, Winthrop Laboratories, New York, N.Y.

D_5/0.25 NS determined by the basic formula. Adjust appropriately for other stock solutions that may be used for maintenance.

Potassium

The maintenance volume is 2 mEq/kg per day. This can be provided by adding 5 mEq to 270 ml of maintenance fluid. (No higher concentration of K^+ should be used routinely.) The maximum amount allowable without an EKG monitor is 40 mEq KCl/liter. Safety depends on minute rate of administration. This must be considered when rapid fluid "pushes" are given.

Vitamins

One-half milliliter of multi-vitamin injection (MVI)* per day in maintenance fluids will provide adequate levels for short-term maintenance.

Blood, Plasma, and Albumin

As required, based on hematocrit and serum protein levels, the following amounts may be given: 20 ml/kg whole blood, plasma, or 5 percent albumin (these are equal to one-fourth of blood volume Æ); 10 ml/kg packed red blood cells; 4 ml/kg 25 percent albumin (salt poor). Any of these volumes are safe to give as a direct push, if no cardiac disease is present.

MEASURED LOSSES OF BODY FLUIDS AND ELECTROLYTES

Volumes

Measure directly and replace milliliter for milliliter.

Electrolyte Content

Gastric suction or vomitus: Sodium, 60 to 75 mEq/liter; chloride: 100 to 150 mEq/liter; potassium: 5 to 20 mEq/liter.The choice here is giving D_5/0.5 NS, replacing sodium but being short of the chloride loss, or giving D_5/NS and thereby an excess of sodium but replacing the chloride. There has been, and still is, much discussion on this matter, but in actual practice the serum electrolytes are better maintained if full chloride replacement is achieved, allowing the kidney to clear excess sodium. Probably the ideal replacement here is D_5/0.5 NS plus 30 to 40 mEq KCl/liter. This provides 77 mEq Na^+, 107 to 117 mEq Cl^-, and 30 to 40 mEq K^+/liter. (See practical tips and examples to clarify this point.)

Gastrointestinal losses distal to the pylorus: Bile, pancreatic juice, fistulous drainage, ileostomy losses, diarrhea, etc. Electrolyte compositions vary

*MVI concentrate, USV Pharmaceutical Corp., Tuckahoe, N.Y.

†Blood volume in a neonate is equal to 8 percent of body weight or 80 ml/kg.[11,18] Thus, one-fourth of blood volume equals 20 ml/kg.

somewhat, but in general the closest inexpensive replacement solution is D_5/RL.

If loss from any part of the gastrointestinal tract persists in excess amounts, actual electrolyte determinations on the fluid are necessary.

A note about evaluation of potassium concentration in serum electrolytes is needed here. Remember that when serum sodium concentration is decreased, potassium shifts out of the cells to offset the positive-ion loss in the vascular space. Therefore, serum potassium may appear to be normal when total body potassium is depleted. When sodium concentration is restored the true potassium deficiency appears. Thus, when the clinical state suggests that potassium should be deficient, and serum sodium is less than normal, adequate potassium replacement is mandatory. This is especially important in a digitalized patient.

THIRD-SPACE SHIFTS

Examples

Examples of third-space shifts include edema, ascites, intraluminal bowel fluids as in ileus or obstruction, intraperitoneal injury secondary to surgical trauma, and opening the previously bypassed capillary beds secondary to vasodilatation after anesthesia and/or surgical trauma. These are all essentially extracellular fluid losses in which these fluid volumes are temporarily unavailable to the vascular system. Some are sequestered; some pass intracellularly.[3]

Volumes

The need for replacement of some volume for such extracellular fluid loss is well accepted; the volumes required are controversial. We accept the need for such replacement, and, since the loss is basically extracellular fluid, we use D_5/RL with or without albumin for the fluid. Neonates respond best if the solution is 5 percent albumin in D_5/RL. The actual volume shifted in any given procedure is immeasurable. Therefore, a pure *guess* is made in writing for such fluid, and the accuracy of the guess is confirmed or rejected by achieving or failing to achieve the desired urine output.

It is very important to grasp here the concept that our goal in optimal fluid management is to refill the vascular space adequately. Fluid shifts to and from any third-space are dynamic, vascular volume being the net result of gains and losses. Attempts to measure third-space per se are fraught with difficulties due to the large number of variables influencing this dynamic fluid state. Although we talk of replacing third-space losses, we are really refilling the vascular space to a level adequate enough to maintain good perfusion as evidenced by urine output. This in turn reflects renal blood flow. To this end we wish to choose a fluid with the least tendency to shift out of the vascular space, ie, one with an adequate osmolality such as D_5/RL or albumin plus D_5/RL.

A simple guideline that has no scientific basis but that has proved helpful in numerous cases over the years for estimating third-space replacement requirements after major intra-abdominal surgery is as follows: For each quadrant of the abdomen either involved in the surgical dissection or affected by the disease process, one-fourth of the maintenance volume of fluid will be required as an additional increment for volume replacement due to third-space shifts. Remember that the fluid chosen must not be a hypotonic "maintenance" type of fluid, but one such as D_5/RL or D_5/RL with 5 percent albumin that is osmotically concentrated. Severe or extensive inflammatory conditions may require one and one-half to twice maintenance as additional volumes.

Examples of various postoperative fluid regimens for a 6-month-old 10-kg infant undergoing various procedures using this guideline are as follows:

Procedure Disease	Maintenance (ml)	Measured Losses	Third-Space Volume
Liver biopsy (1 quadrant)	1000 D_5/0.25 NS	As required	250 D_5/RL
Ladd procedure for malrotation (4 quadrants)	1000 D_5/0.25 NS	As required	1000 D_5/RL + 5% alb
Perforated Meckel's diverticulum with peritonitis (4 quadrants plus severe inflammation)	1000 D_5/0.25 NS	As required	1500–2000 D_5/RL + 5% alb

Once again be cautioned that these are "educated guesses" and must be adjusted appropriately by careful urine output monitoring.

CALCULATION OF DESIRABLE URINE OUTPUT

Metabolic studies show that the urine volume needed to comfortably handle the milliosmolar load of basal metabolism is about 800 to 1000 ml/meter^2/day. This approximates 40 ml/kg per day over a wide range closely enough to make the easier formula useful.[17] This is replaced as free water in the formula for daily maintenance. Since 1200 ml/day is adequate for an adult, when the child reaches 30 kg, he is at maximum output for our purposes.

This urine output is a reasonably optimal level, the achievement of which allows the kidney to function at about one-half maximal concentrating ability and does not overload the patient's cardiovascular system. Remember that it is as important to hold urine down to this level as to strive to achieve this level.

BASIC FACTORS INFLUENCING POSTOPERATIVE FLUID MANAGEMENT: VOLUME RECEPTOR VERSUS OSMORECEPTOR FUNCTIONS

Some further theory and physiologic concepts are important here. First, it is important to realize and remember that we are discussing patients in a dynamic state with regard to vascular volume and extracellular fluid. The injuries and metabolic derangements of the postsurgical/postanesthetic period produce a net loss of vascular volume, inducing a hypovolemia which in turn initiates certain compensatory mechanisms. Among these is the volume receptor monitoring function, which causes the secretion of antidiuretic hormone in the face of volume depletion. If volume restoration is attempted with a hypotonic solution, there is a dilution of serum electrolytes and osmolality. Ordinarily such a dilution would activate osmoreceptors, which would "shut off" antidiuretic hormone and result in excretion of a dilute urine, restoring serum osmolality.[2,19] In the presence of the hypovolemia, however, antidiuretic hormone (ADH) continues to be secreted, a dilute urine cannot be excreted, and thus an osmolar gradient remains between the vascular space and the extravascular fluid, causing a further fall in vascular volume and a dilution of the extravascular osmolality with a net gain of extravascular water.

The other aspect of the compensatory mechanism is the renin–angiotensin–aldosterone system. Any decrease in pressure in the renal juxtaglomerular vessels stimulates renin release. This then promotes angiotensin formation, which stimulates aldosterone release.[20] Aldosterone acts on the renal tubule to facilitate sodium and chloride resorption. In the presence of ADH, this further enhances water resorption from the collecting duct as the osmolality of the medullary area of the kidney is increased.[2] Wright and Gann have shown,[6] however, that a very rapid expansion of the vascular volume, even with a hypotonic solution (1000 ml D_5/water in 20 minutes), will temporarily normalize vascular volume, shutting off the volume receptor stimulus and consequently the antidiuretic hormone secretion and allowing excretion of a dilute urine. Much of this is an osmotic diuretic effect of rapid glucose infusion. This will not permanently restore vascular volume, however, for the osmotic gradient will lead to eventual loss of water to the extravascular tissues as noted above.[21] Hypovolemia will then again stimulate ADH release. For these reasons the use of hypotonic solutions in excess of the amounts calculated for maintenance is contraindicated. Rapid infusions of isotonic solutions will effectively "shut off" the ADH effect.[6]

When blood, plasma, or albumin solutions are given in the presence of hypovolemia and antidiuretic hormone, vascular volume is restored, and there is a net *gain* of intravascular oncotic pressure so that additional fluid may enter the vascular space from the extravascular spaces. When volume is restored, antidiuretic hormone is "shut off" and urine excretion results. Thus, a more permanently restored intravascular volume results.

Transfusion reactions, hepatitis, availability, and cost limit the use of blood, plasma, and albumin for the average patient. When Ringer's lactate is given in the presence of hypovolemia and antidiuretic hormone, the vascular volume is restored. No dilution of intravascular osmolality or electrolyte occurs. There is free diffusion but no osmotic gradient between the extravascular and the vascular spaces, so the vascular volume can be restored and urine excretion achieved without an excessive additional fluid shift to the extravascular tissues.

The above discussion demonstrates that the role of antidiuretic hormone in response to the hypovolemia of surgery and/or trauma is not inappropriate! The secretion of antidiuretic hormone and the corresponding antidiuresis can be overcome by refilling the vascular space. This can be done with hypotonic solutions, but only with very large volumes and at the expense of considerable excess shifting of fluid to the extravascular spaces.[21] This may lead to peripheral, and sometimes interstitial, pulmonary edema.

Solutions with higher osmotic pressures than Ringer's lactate are ideal,[22] but as noted above they have other disadvantages. They should, however, be used when maintenance of an optimal level of intravascular oncotic pressure is particularly important such as in newborns, cardiacs, and cirrhotics. Albumin in Ringer's lactate or saline is the solution of choice here, unless red cells are needed for oxygen-carrying capacity. For the average neonate, D_5/RL containing 5 g percent of salt-poor albumin is the most acceptable solution with regard to all factors. Particularly when intravascular protein and albumin concentrations are known to be or suspected of being depleted, solutions containing albumin are essential.[23] Otherwise, even full electrolyte solutions such as D_5/NS or D_5/RL may shift out of the vascular space due to the protein oncotic gradient.

Another important consideration in line with the above discussion is that of always giving D_5/RL or D_5/RL with albumin as the *initial* postoperative fluid and continuing this until an adequate urine output is well established.

Only thus can we be certain that vascular volume is restored and that antidiuretic hormone will not interfere with proper utilization of the more hypotonic solutions when they are added. If this consideration is ignored and hypovolemia does exist, dilute solutions will be retained, a net shift into the extravascular tissues along the oncotic gradient may occur, and edema will result. This may be of minimal consequence in the average patient, but in a patient with pulmonary insufficiency, sepsis, or "shock lung," this edema in the interstitial tissues of the lung may increase alveolar–capillary block and severely increase pulmonary insufficiency.[23,24]

Recently, the issue of when to use albumin has been much debated in the literature.[24–26] It has been shown that, whenever capillary integrity breaks down, albumin "leaks" into the perivascular tissues, causing a detrimental "reverse" oncotic gradient.[27] When pulmonary capillary integrity is disturbed, as in septic shock lung, albumin should be avoided until capillary integrity is restored. In other situations, particularly in the neonate with his tendency to deplete intravascular albumin rapidly, albumin may be very beneficial in preventing fluid shifts to the pulmonary interstitium.[23,24,28]

ASSOCIATED DYSFUNCTIONS: CARDIAC AND HEPATIC

Cardiac, renal, and hepatic dysfunctions create added difficulties in fluid management. One obviously cannot disregard the effects of these dysfunctions on replacement problems. Neither, on the other hand, can vascular volume replacement needs be disregarded because other problems exist coincidentally. Just as some modifications of fluid programs may be necessary, so, too, one must be ready and willing to use drugs to improve cardiac, hepatic, and renal function to enable these organs to function optimally in the face of volume deficits. There is no place here for the purist who refuses to digitalize a heart that is functioning subnormally in the face of a serious hypovolemic or septic state just because either it has functioned adequately previously, or no diagnostic label has as yet been pinned on the cardiac malfunction!

Certainly, guidance and consultation with knowledgeable members of the pediatric staff are mandatory when serious multisystems dysfunctions are present, but some idea of the dosage and agents of importance in handling such problems should be in the surgeon's armamentarium as well. Suggestions are presented in the appendix to this section.

When dealing with severe liver dysfunction, as in biliary atresia or cirrhosis following neonatal hepatitis, as well as in some cardiac insufficiency situations, diuretics may aid considerably in both preoperative preparation and postoperative management. The following are examples:

1. Neonatal bowel obstruction associated with decompensating cardiac anomalies. A patient, fully digitalized, still requires major fluid replacement volumes, but circulatory insufficiency persists as evidenced by peripheral edema and pulmonary insufficiency.
2. An otherwise normal cardiac status in a patient with severe gram-negative sepsis and shock. Attempts to restore volume have produced further cardiac decompensation with pulmonary and peripheral edema. Digitalization has been accomplished, but no diuresis has occurred yet.
3. Liver decompensation with cirrhosis and ascites preoperatively or developing postoperatively in patients with high-volume fluid requirements secondary to extensive surgery; also in shock states secondary to variceal hemorrhage in the same patients. In these instances high-volume fluid replacement is necessary, but the patient's circulatory system will not handle the loads efficiently. The intravascular oncotic pressure is reduced due to low levels of plasma proteins, especially albumin, and sodium excretion is reduced by the high level of circulating aldosterone.

In extreme cases, diuresis and continued fluid administration may be required simultaneously! In general, however, restoration of normal circulatory dynamics is impossible in cirrhotics until adequate improvement in intravascular oncotic pressure is achieved by improving serum albumin and protein levels. Repeated paracenteses will only cause further ascitic accumulations and further losses of body proteins. A combination of albumin administration with careful diuresis may be ideal in the acute stages. Example 3 below outlines some important facets of the management of such patients.

Diuretics may significantly improve circulatory function. When faced with the chronic liver failure and ascites of the cirrhotic infant, the long-term use of spironolactone* (3mg/kg per 24 hours per ora) and hydrochlorothiazide† (2 mg/kg per 24 hours) is ideal, but for some acute problems it is of little use. Ethacrinic acid‡ or furosemide§ are the agents of choice for the acute diuretic problem. Dosage is 1 mg/kg up to the adult dose of 50 mg. With any of these agents, careful monitoring of serum electrolytes and weight is important, and maintenance of adequate K^+ levels must be ensured.

*Aldactone, Searle & Co., San Juan, Puerto Rico.
†HydroDiuril, Merck, Sharp & Dohme, West Point, Pa.
‡Edecrin, Merck, Sharp & Dohme, West Point, Pa.
§Lasix, Hoechst-Roussel Pharmaceuticals Inc., Somerville, N.J.

If oral alimentation is possible, potassium may be given as potassium gluconate (20 mEq potassium per 15 ml).* Remember the maintenance figure of 2 to 3 mEq/kg per day in prescribing.

For intravenous potassium replacement direct addition of KCl to the reservoir is indicated. No more than 40 mEq/1000 ml or 10 mEq/250 ml should ordinarily be administered without EKG and serum electrolyte monitoring.

The availability of dopamine† has made many of these circulatory deficiency states easier to manage. Dopamine has an inotropic effect on the myocardium, improving cardiac output and circulatory efficiency as well as renal and probably mesenteric perfusion. Thus, the benefits of digitalization are achieved without the risks of bradycardia and arrhythmia. Simultaneously improved renal perfusion leads to more urine output, better body fluid balance, and decreased fluid retention without the risk of electrolyte wastage that frequently results from the administration of furosemide. Example 4 below illustrates a hypothetical case study in which the use of pharmacotherapeutic agents is illustrated.

With this theoretical background at hand, one can now proceed to manage postoperative fluid requirements with careful consideration of the following basic categories: (a) Maintenance limited to calculated values, avoiding excessive amounts of hypotonic fluids; (b) measurable losses replaced volume for volume with appropriate solutions; and (c) third-space losses replaced by using urine output as an indicator of adequate vascular volume restoration.

PRACTICAL GUIDELINES FOR FLUID MANAGEMENT

1. All fluid orders for the ensuing 24 hours are to be written in the early morning after evaluating the current status of the patient. Either cancel remaining orders from the previous 24 hours or make clear that they are to be included as the first part of the new series, clearly indicating that any change in rate applies to these items as well. In cardiac, severely ill, and early postoperative patients check more often, at least every 4 hours.

2. All patients should be weighed at least once daily. Weighing is of little value in the immediate postoperative period, however, because if third-space shifts are adequately replaced, weight gain is expected.

3. No child should be exposed to a reservoir containing more fluid than he can tolerate as a rapid "push." A volume control chamber‡ should be in-

*Kaon Elixer, Warren-Teed Pharmaceuticals Inc., Columbus, Ohio.
†Intropin, Arnar-Stone Laboratories Inc., Mount Prospect, Ill.
‡Soluset, Abbott Laboratories, Chicago, Ill.

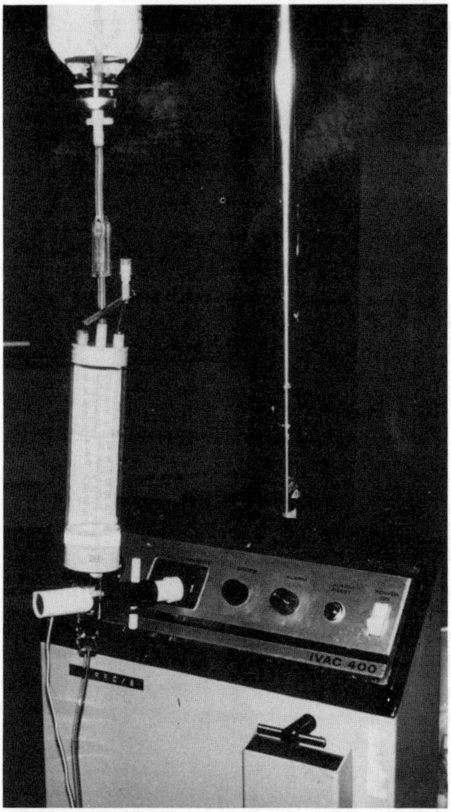

FIG. 1. A safety chamber and an infusion pump interposed between the resevoir and the patient prevent accidental fluid overload.

terposed between the main fluid reservoir and the patient (Fig. 1). Never expose a child to a reservoir equal to more than one-fourth of his blood volume.

4. When changing rates, be certain to indicate which items are included and call the attention of the nurse to the change.

5. With rare exceptions all parenteral fluids should contain at least 5% dextrose, and all children on parenteral feeding should receive vitamins daily. Premature infants and many newborns require 10% dextrose and supplemental albumin or plasma.

6. Establishing intravenous lines in young children is time-consuming, difficult, and often frustrating. Protect them with careful taping, splinting, and retaping as necessary, and avoid phlebitis by adding 1 unit of heparin to each milliliter of fluid in all lines. This is a perfectly safe dose even in a preoperative patient. Check the condition of the extremity on rounds daily, and discontinue the line when any evidence of phlebitis or infiltration is noted.

7. With neonates and small infants in hypovolemic shock, "pump priming" is essential to restore circulating volume quickly. This is safely done by pushing in 20 ml/kg (one-fourth of the blood volume) of electrolyte or colloid solution in a well-established IV. This amount is not figured into maintenance or replacement fluid amounts or composition.

8. Use an infusion pump for small volume rates (less than 10 ml/hour).

9. When the fluid problems are serious and a careful monitoring and adjustment of rate is desired, you may order a set rate and then write: "Increase or decrease the rate in increments of X ml/hour to keep q1h urine output between Y and Z ml/hour. If correction is not obtained after two such changes, call MD." This will allow the nurses to make ongoing hourly changes and maintain a smoother fluid management program.

10. Volume maximums for volume control chambers* are as follows: 2000-g infant, 25-ml increments; newborns, full-sized, 50-ml increments; infants 4 kg and over, 100-ml increments. In general, the increment may not exceed one-fourth of the infant's blood volume. These are the amounts to put in the chamber at one time and thereby the maximum accidental infusion to which the child is at risk.

11. To avoid multiple repetitions of additives to each ordered increment, write as follows:

Stock A: 270 ml D_5/0.25 NS + 5 mEq KCl + 5 ml

Calcium Gluconate + 2.5 ml MVI + 270 units heparin

Stock B: 270 ml D_5/RL + 5 mEq KCl + 270 units heparin

(1) 50 ml A; (2) 50 ml A; (3) 50 ml B; (4) 50 ml B; etc.

These stock solutions should be made up fresh each day and must be rewritten at the top of each order sheet.

12. All intravenous antibiotics are given into the intravenous line. You may order 5 to 10 ml D_5/0.25 NS to dissolve and carry in each dose. Particularly in neonates and infants you must take account of this volume, reducing maintenance appropriately, or you will give more than required maintenance amounts and may severely overload the premature infant. Remember to adjust for the sodium or potassium concentration of various antibiotics. Direct intravenous push of medications is preferred, however, since this avoids excess fluid loads. Avoid rapid pushes of ampicillin, however, as this may cause convulsions. When one or more additional monitoring lines, such as arterial cannulas or central venous lines, are in place, the fluids used to infuse or flush these lines must be considered in planning maintenance and replacement volumes. Failure to do so may lead to serious overloads in the small infant.

*Soluset, Abbott Laboratories, Chicago, Ill.

EXAMPLES OF PARENTERAL FLUID AND ELECTROLYTE MANAGEMENT

EXAMPLE 1

A 4-kg, 3-week-old infant, is one day postoperative resection and ileoileostomy for malrotation with volvulus. Nasogastric suction for the previous 24 hours, 75 ml; hematocrit is 40 percent; urine output for the previous 24 hours is 120 ml.

Maintenance

Water: (100 ml $-3\times$ age in years) (Weight in kg) $=$ 100 ml $\times$ 4 kg $=$ 400 ml

Sodium and chloride: 3 mEq/kg $=$ 12 mEq

Potassium: 2 mEq/kg $=$ 8 mEq

The requirement is satisfied by 400 ml D_5/0.25 NS +8 mEq KCl.

Nasogastric Replacement

Water: 75 ml

Sodium at 60 to 75 mEq/liter $=$ 5 mEq

Chloride at 100 to 150 mEq/liter $=$ 8 to 10 mEq

Potassium at 10 to 30 mEq/liter $=$ 3 mEq

The requirement is satisfied by 75 ml D_5/0.5 NS plus 3 mEq KCl. This provides Na^+, 5.7 mEq; Cl^-, 5.7 + 3 mEq = 8.7 mEq; K^+, 3 mEq.

Third-Space Loss

Fluid: D_5/RL or plasma

The amount of fluid needed is a *guess*. To arrive at a reasonable guess, think about your adult experience and utilize the previously suggested abdominal quadrant guideline. If an adult requires 1500 ml of maintenance and for a procedure such as a bowel obstruction you would give an additional 1500 to 2000 ml D_5/RL for third-space shifts, relate this experience to the child's maintenance as follows:

$$\frac{\text{Adult third space}}{\text{Adult maintenance}} = \frac{\text{Child third space}}{\text{Child maintenance}}$$

$$\frac{1500\text{ ml}}{1500\text{ ml}} = \frac{400\text{ ml}}{400\text{ ml}} \qquad \text{or } 1 \times \text{maintenance}$$

This is the guess for D_5/RL needs for this situation. Similarly, in a situation in which you would give an adult 750 ml of D_5/RL for third-space losses, or one-half his maintenance, you can estimate the child's need at one-half his maintenance so that the 4-kg infant in question would get an additional 200 ml of D_5/RL beyond his maintenance and measured losses. Thus, in this example we would give

75 ml D_5/0.5 NS + 3 mEq KCl
400 ml D_5/0.25 NS + 8 mEq KCl
400 ml D_5/RL
875 ml fluid

A total of 875 ml fluid in 24 hours would require a rate of about 37 ml/hour. Therefore, we would order the fluids to start running at this rate and watch the urine output.

Urine output should be 40 ml/kg per day = 160 ml/day for this 4-kg infant, or about 7 ml/hour. If the urine output is less than 7 ml/hour, we have guessed too little third-space loss and must add more D_5/RL or plasma. If it is more than 7 ml/hour, we have guessed too much third-space loss and must therefore give less D_5/RL or plasma. Notice that this has no bearing on the previously calculated maintenance and measured loss amounts.

If a few of the increments of D_5/RL are always placed at the end of the day's fluids, slowing the intravenous rate will result in elimination of some of the ordered D_5/RL, effectively reducing the excess. If the intravenous rate must be increased because the urine output is too little, more fluids will have to be added to cover the 24-hour period and this added fluid will almost always be D_5/RL or plasma, since again it was the allowance for third-space losses that was most likely originally miscalculated.

Another frequent source of miscalculation, however, is in nasogastric losses. Frequently, the rest of the day after surgery the loss may be minimal. Consequently, measured loss replacements would be low. During the subsequent 24 hours, this volume often increases markedly, in which case the fluid needs would be greater because of this and not because of miscalculated third-space needs.

EXAMPLE 2

A 5-year-old, 20-kg male had a splenectomy three days ago for idiopathic thrombocytopenic purpura. Nasogastric loss for the previous 24 hours was 800 ml; urine output was 1200 ml.

Maintenance

Water: (100 ml − 3 × 5) (20) = 85 × 20 = 1700 ml, which we would round back to the 1500 ml that we consider to be adult maintenance.

Sodium and chloride: 3 mEq/kg up to adult maintenance of 45 to 60 mEq
Potassium: 2 mEq/kg up to adult 40 mEq

The requirement is satisfied by 1500 ml D_5/0.25 NS + 40 mEq KCl.

Nasogastric replacement

Water: 800 ml
Sodium: 60 to 75 mEq/liter (75) = 60 mEq in 800 ml
Chloride: 100 to 150 mEq/liter (105) = 84 mEq in 800 ml
Potassium: 30 mEq/liter = 24 mEq in 800 ml
Therefore, replace with

800 ml D_5/0.5 NS + 24 mEq KCl
= 60 mEq Na^+
= 84 mEq Cl
= 24 mEq K^+

Third-Space Loss

Since by the third day third-space losses not only are decreasing, but may be actually returning to the functional and vascular compartments, a look at the previous day's urine output will determine this need. If it is equal to the desired amount, no third-space fluid is calculated but may need to be added later if urine volume falls. If it exceeds considerably the desired level, not only is no D_5/RL given, but less maintenance may be required, since fluid is entering the functional compartments from within and will thus maintain the vascular volume. Thus, one might give only 1500 ml total fluid since yesterday's urine of 1200 ml far exceeds the desired 800 ml (40 ml/kg). If this is done, however, as much of the nasogastric NaCl loss should be replaced as possible. There is, of course, already excess sodium aboard in the third-space fluid that has been replaced by D_5/RL on previous days.

EXAMPLE 3

A more difficult problem is that of a child with liver disease undergoing extensive surgery. Consider the case of a 10-year-old boy weighing 30 kg with a history of neonatal hepatitis followed by repeated episodes of variceal bleeding beginning at age 5 years and becoming increasingly severe and more frequent. With each episode, liver function tests become abnormal, showing evidence of chronic liver impairment with elevated serum bilirubin, SGOT, and alkaline phosphatase; depressed serum proteins and clotting factors; and the development of ascites.

Because of the increasing frequency of the serious variceal hemorrhages, a portocaval shunt is performed after three weeks of intensive preparation in the hospital with good nutrition, intravenous albumin supplements, therapeutic vitamin levels, transfusion to hematocrit of 41 percent, and correction of prothrombin time to 87 percent with intramuscular vitamin K. Nevertheless, at surgery, 200 ml of ascitic fluid is removed from the peritoneal cavity. Blood loss of 1000 ml is replaced.

At 8:00 A.M. the next day, you must order his next 24 hours of intravenous intake. Consider the following:

1. Maintenance is defined as usual.
2. Replace nasogastric losses as usual.
3. Major differences will involve the following:
   a. High levels of circulating aldosterone will produce sodium retention.
   b. There will be decreased intravascular oncotic pressure.
   c. High-resistance liver circuit tends to reform ascites through intrahepatic sinusoids.
   d. Surgery, anesthesia, and shunt of portal blood tend to further injure liver.
4. We can assume, therefore, that:
   a. Salt will be poorly handled.
   b. Intravascular oncotic pressure will tend to fall.
   c. Potassium levels will be critical for their role in acid–base balance, which affects the dissociation equation of ammonia.[29]
5. In figuring third-space losses we should, therefore:
   a. Minimize them by maintaining intravascular oncotic pressure high with blood and plasma or albumin.
   b. Keep hematocrit above 40 percent.
   c. Give frequent 20 ml/kg pushes of 5 percent albumin or give 4 ml/kg of 25 percent albumin (salt poor).

d. After the above is accomplished, give D_5/RL as needed to maintain urine output, but accept reduced level of about 25 to 30 ml/kg per day to insure against volume overload.

e. Monitor urine and central venous pressure (CVP) and electrolytes.

f. If CVP and electrolytes are within normal limits and urine output is low after the above fluid administration, try diuretics to offset the increased levels of circulating aldosterone, but carefully maintain K^+ levels by giving optimal replacement.

EXAMPLE 4

A 2200-g female infant is born as twin B and appears well at birth. Apgar score is 8/10. The child does well for two days, then becomes distended and vomits bile-stained gastric content. Distention progresses rapidly; the child becomes dehydrated and lethargic. Color and tone are poor. Urine output falls to zero. An upper gastrointestinal study shows an apparent obstruction in the upper jejunum with gas in bowel beyond this point down to the rectum. A meconium stool is guaiac positive.

After resuscitation, the child is taken to surgery, where a segment of mid-small bowel is found to be perforated from necrotizing enterocolitis. The segment is resected and an end-to-end anastomosis is performed in well-vascularized, normal-appearing bowel. The peritoneal cavity is extensively cleaned mechanically and lavaged with copious amounts of warmed saline solution to rid it of most of the spilled bowel contents. A radial artery cannula and a subclavian central venous catheter are established.

During surgery the child received 90 ml D_5/RL, 10 ml 25 percent salt-poor albumin, and 50 ml whole blood. Blood loss was 20 ml. Outline the postoperative fluids you would give this child as follows:

Maintenance

$$(100 - 3 \times \text{age in years})(\text{weight in kg}) = 100 \times 2.2 = 220 \text{ ml}$$

Measured Losses

Blood adequately replaced.

Third-Space Loss

Perforation and peritonitis require 1.5 to 2 times maintenance. Therefore, third-space loss is 330 to 440 ml. Since intraoperative fluid management was quite good, we would hold to the lower figure. Therefore, begin D_5/RL with 5 percent albumin at rate to get in

$$\begin{array}{rl} & 330 \text{ ml third-space guess} \\ + & \underline{220 \text{ ml maintenance}} \\ & 550 \text{ ml in 24 hours} \\ = & 23 \text{ ml/hour} \end{array}$$

Continue D_5/RL with albumin until urine output reaches 3 to 4 ml/hour and stabilizes (40 ml/kg per day = 88 ml/day = 3 to 4 ml/hour). Then begin to add in some D_5/0.25 NS alternating with remaining D_5/RL.

Question: What other factors must be considered in managing this child?

Necrotizing enterocolitis with perforation and peritonitis is a severe septic challenge. In addition to antibiotics and the careful peritoneal cleaning, a two for one exchange transfusion was performed with fresh whole blood. This was done with the hope of washing out some of the toxins and offsetting the frequent tendency in these children to succumb to disseminated intravascular coagulopathy.[30,31]

Question: What other pathophysiologic problems may arise?

As sepsis progresses, it may depress myocardial contractility, lessen circulatory efficiency, interfere with pulmonary capillary integrity, and cause inappropriate ADH secretion. Any or all of these may decrease renal blood flow, glomerular filtration rate, and urine output. Thus, excess fluid volumes may be administered and the child may be overloaded without ever showing the appropriate urinary response.

Here the CVP line is invaluable, for it will show when hypovolemia is corrected or indicate circulatory inefficiency secondary to sepsis. Initially, the CVP read 17. A repeat chest x-ray revealed the catheter in the right ventricle. After the catheter was withdrawn 4 cm, the reading was zero. The post-exchange hematocrit was 37 percent. Forty-four milliliters of whole blood were given (20 ml/kg) and fluids administered as planned. The CVP gradually rose to 8 cm water with only 1 to 2 ml urine output per hour.

The next morning the serum albumin was 2.1 mg%. Albumin was added to all solutions to make 5 percent albumin concentrations, and twice daily "pushes" of albumin, 4 ml/kg, were given. The serum albumin rose to 4.4 mg%. Urine output remained low. The child gained weight and became edematous. Central venous pressure rose to 13 cm water.

Question: What is now happening?

Although the child has not succumbed to overwhelming sepsis (platelet count remains 250,000), she probably has some deficiency in cardiac output or a persistent "inappropriate" ADH secretion secondary to sepsis. Blood culture grew *Klebsiella* sensitive to the antibiotics being administered. Urine output remained low even after concentrated albumin injections.

Question: What are the treatment options?

Digoxin would improve myocardial function and would probably result in increased renal perfusion and diuresis, but arrhythmias might result, and overdosage could produce bradycardia. Furosemide would produce diuresis rapidly but would not sustain improved circulation dynamics. Dopamine would improve both myocardial contractility and renal perfusion.

Initially furosemide was chosen, since CVP was elevated, body weight increased, and serum electrolytes elevated (Na^+, 147; Cl, 113; K^+, 5.3). This resulted in a transient diuresis of 45 ml urine over 4 hours, but output again fell. The CVP decreased to 10 cm water.

A dopamine drip was instituted at 5 μg/minute. Urine output rose to 8 ml/hour; CVP fell to 7 cm water, and the diuresis was sustained. After 36 hours the dopamine was gradually tapered and discontinued. The child sustained the diuresis with dopamine and weight returned to 2200 g.

TOTAL PARENTERAL NUTRITION (TPN)

INTRODUCTION

The need for and possibility of maintaining patients in positive nitrogen balance and good long-term nutritional status by parenteral means have fascinated and frustrated surgeons for many decades. Much of the groundwork had already been provided,[32] some of it in their own laboratories, [33,34] when Dudrick, Wilmore, and Rhoads combined a high-calorie mixture of glucose and protein hydrolysates with the central venous catheter to give the misnomered "hyperalimentation" to the medical world.[35—37]

Since pediatric surgery provided some of the first few human subjects on whom the new treatment was carried out,[36,38] it is only fitting that pediatric surgery, as well as general pediatrics, should be a principal beneficiary of the new technique. Properly applied, it has contributed magnificently to the survival of infants previously hopelessly lost, but it is fraught with hazards and complications and requires knowledgeable and experienced application.

INDICATIONS FOR USE IN PEDIATRIC SURGERY

Total intravenous alimentation should never be used when a usable gastrointestinal route is available, as its risks are too great, especially in the neonate and young infant. However, when temporary unavailability of the gastrointestinal tract threatens to lead to death in a child with a correctable lesion, its contributions to survival are immeasurable. A reasonably sure end point for the gastrointestinal nonavailability must be foreseen, however. To undertake parenteral nutrition in a child with little or no hope of eventual normal alimentation is a tragedy of suffering for all concerned as well as an inexcusable cost in terms of personnel time and hospitalization expense. Thus, a child whose total small intestine is destroyed by disease, vascular accident, or volvulus from malrotation should never be started on this therapy. Wilmore found that resumption of gastrointestinal alimentation with progress in development was unlikely if less than 30 cm of small bowel remained without the ileocecal valve.[39] One child with an intact ileocecal process progressed satisfactorily with 15 cm of additional small intestine.

CONDITIONS THAT FREQUENTLY REQUIRE AND BENEFIT FROM TOTAL PARENTERAL ALIMENTATION

These conditions include the following:

1. Giant omphaloceles and gastroschises requiring staged repairs (Fig. 2)

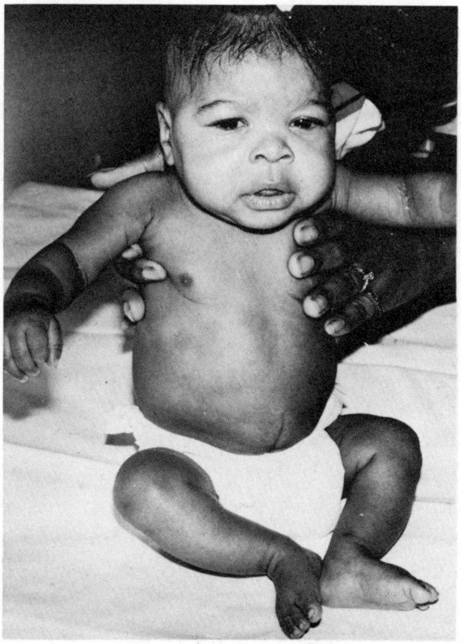

FIG. 2. This 3-month-old baby was maintained on total parenteral nutrition for five weeks while reduction of her gastroschisis was accomplished (see Figs. 67 and 68).

2. Multiple congenital atresias with or without short bowel syndrome
3. Necrotizing enterocolitis, acutely and during prolonged recovery, and correction of secondary atresias, stenoses, and fistulas
4. Esophageal atresias with tracheoesophageal fistulas while awaiting definitive repair, particularly when aspiration pneumonia delays surgery
5. In utero and neonatal perforations
6. Complications of tumor radiotherapy
7. Small bowel fistulas from any cause

PREFERRED CANNULATION SITES IN INFANTS

The most widely used sites are the internal jugular veins reached through a supraclavicular incision and using a tunneling technique to achieve catheter exit in the scalp.[40] This approach is unimaginative and potentially hazardous since ligation of the deep jugulars bilaterally may lead to hydrocephalus or superior vena cava syndrome.

An attempt should always be made to cannulate the external jugulars first, and frequently this can be done even in neonates. If the internal veins must be utilized, a 7/0 silk purse string suture in the anterior surface obviates ligation and may preserve flow.

Other sites are the antecubital veins, particularly the basilic. This can often be cannulated percutaneously with an 18-gauge percutaneous plastic cannula with the following catheter threaded centrally.* Adjustments can be made under fluoroscopic control. The Castro-y-Juevo cyclodialysis spatula is a valuable aid in cannulation when incisional exposure of the vein is undertaken.

If one has sufficient experience with the use of subclavian puncture, this technique can be utilized in older infants[41,42] and now promises to be more easily and safely achieved in newborns with the advent of the plastic cannulation system* (see Figs. 14 and 15).

We have required that our residents be accomplished at peripheral cannulation in infants, have extensive experience with adult subclavian cannulation, and be supervised in about 12 procedures before allowing them to perform subclavian puncture in infants independently. Over 100 subclavian cannulations have been performed for infants on our service without a significant complication. Most have weighed less than 2500 g, and many have been under 1000 g.

As with any centrally placed line, confirmation of position by easy blood

*Argyle Intramedicut Catheter, Sherwood Medical Industries, Inc., St. Louis, Mo.

return and x-ray localization is mandatory (see Fig. 16). In addition, injection of 1 ml of contrast medium ensures that intraluminal position is obtained.

COMPLICATIONS

Sepsis far outdistances all other complications and consequences.[43] Careful aseptic methods are required at all phases of insertion and maintenance of the line. These factors are discussed in the next part of this chapter (pp. 27–31; 56–60).

Improper placement may lead to extravasation, hemorrhage, pneumothorax, hemothorax, or hydrothorax with attendant risks of mediastinal shifts, ventilatory embarrassment, and cardiovascular compromise.

Candida sepsis is the most potentially significant infection.[43,44] Widespread candidiasis is damaging and frequently lethal. Vigilance is required for recognition and early treatment.

Removal of the line is almost a sine qua non of treatment for sepsis. Studies have shown that a properly cared for system rarely initiates the infection but tends to harbor organisms entering through other portals.[45,46]

PRINCIPLES OF PARENTERAL ALIMENTATION

By this time the amount of literature on this subject is overwhelming, yet many basic questions, such as the ideal composition of the solution, remain unanswered. The essentials of administration, as presently understood, are as follows:

1. The basic solution is formed by mixing approximately 20 percent dextrose solution with 5 percent protein hydrolysate or free amino acids in some proportion to provide a solution with approximately 1 cal/ml. This is combined with maintenance electrolytes, heparin, and vitamins including vitamin K. Appropriate additions of folate and B_{12} must be made.
2. No trace minerals or essential fatty acids are provided by the basic formula. The neonate especially requires fatty acids for myelinization of neurons. At present, fresh frozen plasma given twice weekly is the easiest source of supply for these. Intravenous fat emulsion* supplementation is now available and should ease this problem.[47]
3. Electrolyte content must be adjusted for abnormal losses by adding appropriate additional amounts to the basic formula.
4. Insulin levels quickly compensate for the high calorie load. Additional stimulation to β cells is provided by the amino acids such as leucine in the protein hydrolysate. Adjustment generally is rapid enough that exogenous

*Intralipid, 10 percent intravenous fat emulsion, Cutler Laboratories, Inc., Berkeley, Calif.

insulin rarely is required.[40] Glycosuria recurring after stabilization, however, may be the first sign of sepsis.

The guidelines for formula content in the article by Heird and Winters[48] will aid in developing an appropriate solution.

SUGGESTIONS FOR MANAGEMENT OF TOTAL PARENTERAL NUTRITION

SOLUTION ADMINISTRATION

Most full-term infants and older children will tolerate initiation at maintenance fluid volumes with full caloric solution (1 cal/ml). This equals 100 ml/kg per day for infants 7 days to 1 year of age. This must be considerably modified for small premature infants. [48,49] Initial glucose load should be halved and protein begun at 1 g/kg per day.

Older infants and children may be started at full maintenance by the formula (100 ml − 3× age in years) (weight in kilograms).

These levels should be continued for three to four days. When the child has stabilized on this regimen, 10 percent increments of additional fluid per day should be added every three to four days until a sustained weight gain is achieved. This usually requires about 125 cal/ kg per day.

The addition of albumin (25 percent salt poor) at 4 ml/kg per day as a supplemental intravenous injection will greatly facilitate the child's ability to tolerate these fluid volumes during the first few weeks of therapy. This is especially true for the child in moderate to severe negative nitrogen balance when therapy is initiated. The albumin functions to increase the intravascular oncotic pressure.[26,28]

Twice weekly increments of 20 ml/kg of fresh frozen plasma will provide trace elements and essential fatty acids.[48] Albumin need not be given on the days plasma is administered. Without essential fatty acids, proper myelinization of nerve tissue may be impaired. The availability of intravenous lipid emulsions* should simplify the problem of providing needed fat substances.[47,50]

Ongoing electrolyte losses should be corrected by having pharmacy add appropriate additional increments to the base formula.

MONITORING

Until the child has achieved stability on the regimen (usually 48 to 72 hours), twice daily blood glucose levels and glucose determinations on all

*Intralipid, 10 percent intravenous fat emulsion, Cutler Laboratories, Berkeley, Calif.

urine volumes should be performed. Serum and urinary osmolality determinations would be ideal, if readily available. Almost all children tolerate the above program without need for corrective therapy, however.[40]

If the urine glucose is 4+ or greater, insulin may be added at 0.5 unit/50 ml formula. This is rarely necessary and can usually be discontinued after a short time. The Boston Children's group has shown that even at 4+, less than 1 percent administered glucose is lost in the urine.[40]

Once the child is stable, glucose and electrolyte determinations can be determined every three days to correspond with blood culture and dressing change routines.

Imbalances of calcium, phosphorus, magnesium, and ammonia may occur and should be routinely monitored.[48] Obstructive jaundice is another complication of prolonged parenteral alimentation, so monitoring of bilirubin, alkaline phosphatase, and liver enzymes should be programmed.[51]

If sudden dislodgement or obstruction causes unplanned discontinuance of the parenteral regimen, great care must be exercised to recognize and treat an acute hypoglycemia that may result.

Daily platelet counts will provide the best indication of any impending sepsis. Any marked fall should be viewed with great suspicion. Once sepsis is confirmed, the line must be discontinued and provisions made for peripheral fluid administration.

The routine blood cultures obtained every three days (see the section below on nursing care procedures for TPN) may prove invaluable if and when sepsis supervenes.

NURSING CARE PROCEDURES FOR TOTAL PARENTERAL ALIMENTATION OF INFANTS

The following outline is our present procedure for the management of TPN lines in the intensive care nursery at Duke University Medical Center:

I. Catheter Placement and Stabilization

  A. The catheter is placed in the operating room by the pediatric surgical service under sterile operating conditions. Only local anesthesia is used unless the child is undergoing a concomitant operative procedure.

  B. The catheter used is Intramedicut, a polyvinyl chloride catheter with radiopaque marker.

  C. Generally, all catheters are placed percutaneously via the subclavian vein and advanced into the superior vena cava.

    1. Only on rare occasions is incisional placement via the jugular vein required.

2. No "tunneling" is required when the percutaneous method is used.

D. The catheters are sutured in place at the puncture site and 1 cm distal to the puncture site with silk sutures.

E. Proper catheter placement is determined by:

1. Successful free aspiration of *venous* blood.

2. Instillation of contrast media into the catheter to rule out extravascular placement or extravasation.

3. An anteroposterior portable x-ray to delineate catheter position and check for any inadvertent pneumothorax (obtained in the operating room).
Note: Since the catheter is radiopaque, its position can be monitored at any time by portable chest x-ray.

F. The catheter is then taped in place appropriately. Either previously prepared TPN solution or a temporary solution of heparinized electrolytes is started.

G. The baby is returned to the ward directly from the operating room.

II. Catheter Maintenance

A. The catheter is attached to a constant infusion pump and is not used to withdraw blood, infuse other solutions, or inject medications except under special circumstances defined in point III below.

B. Stopcocks are not to be used with parenteral alimentation catheters.

C. The day-charge nurse along with other previously trained personnel provide care for the system as follows:

1. Each day the solution, all tubing, and the filter are renewed down to the catheter itself.

2. When the catheter is being disconnected, it should be clamped with a small rubber shod clamp to prevent air embolism. The rubber prevents damage to the plastic tube.

3. The dressing and taping are inspected and either reinforced or changed as needed.

4. On Monday, Wednesday, and Friday complete dressing change, wound care, and retaping are accomplished as follows:

a. Remove cross-strips of tape holding loop of catheter.

b. Remove "upside-down" strip of tape from beneath catheter.

c. Remove long strip of tape from chest and dressing but do not remove this strip from catheter itself—cut off excess tape.

d. Remove dressing carefully to avoid dislodging catheter.

e. Check integrity of sutures; call surgery to resuture pro re nata.

f. Using aseptic technique, defat puncture site and surrounding skin with acetone.

g. Prep the area with Betadine solution and allow Betadine to dry.

h. Apply Betadine ointment in limited amount to puncture site and sutures.

i. Apply tincture of benzoin to skin.

j. Apply 2×2 or spot dressing and tape thoroughly in place.

k. Reapply one long strip of waterproof tape extending length of catheter across dressing and well onto skin of chest.

l. Apply "upside-down" strip of tape.

m. Further tape cross-strips as appropriate.

n. Clamp catheter with rubber-protected mosquito hemostat to prevent air embolism.

o. Disconnect line, draw appropriate studies, flush line thoroughly, and attach new connecting lines, filter, and fresh solution.

p. Unclamp catheter and insure flow.

D. Send the used system components to bacteriology for culture of both sides of system.

E. All solutions run through central lines must contain 1 unit heparin per milliliter solution.

III. Exceptions to General Rules Regarding Catheter Care.

A. Antibiotics

1. When antibiotics are being given for sepsis thought to be associated with the line, they should be given through the line.

2. Injection should be into a T-connector nipple prepped with Betadine.

B. Blood cultures

1. On Monday, Wednesday and Friday, when the entire system and dressing are changed, a blood culture should be drawn through the line; additional blood may be drawn up in the syringe for other studies at this time.

2. The system should then be thoroughly flushed with heparinized solution before the new tubing is attached (see point II,C,4,o).

C. Central venous pressure monitoring

1. Frequently, babies after major surgical procedures require CVP monitoring. These lines are not used for parenteral nutrition simultaneously. Five percent dextrose in electrolyte solutions heparinized with 1 unit heparin per milliliter of solution is generally used.

2. Pressure readings by direct readout with a continuous infusion system are preferable to manual monitoring with stopcock and tube column.

D. Conversion of CVP line to TPN line. Once the need for CVP monitoring has passed, if use of the central line for TPN is desirable, the following is done:

1. Change the tubing and dressing in the usual fashion, reestablishing a closed, filtered system using heparinized 5 percent dextrose/electrolyte solution.

2. Discontinue all monitoring systems connected to the line.

3. Draw a blood culture through the line.

4. If the blood culture shows no growth after 48 hours and the baby shows no sign of infection, TPN is then added to the system.

E. Sepsis. If a child develops signs of sepsis while a central line for TPN is in place, the following procedure should be instituted:

1. Stop the TPN solution.
2. Run 5 percent dextrose/electrolyte solution with heparin, 1 unit/ml.
3. Draw a blood culture through the line.
4. Institute antibiotic therapy through the line.
5. Monitor platelets, vital signs, and general condition.
6. If child improves, reculture line daily, and if organism clears resume TPN.
7. If child worsens or bacteremia persists discontinue line and wait 48 hours after bacteremia clears before instituting a new line.

CHAPTER 2

PRINCIPLES OF GENERAL CARE FOR THE NEWBORN

TRANSPORTATION AND INITIAL CARE

TRANSPORTATION

Prior Preparation

Depending on the familiarity of the referring institution with newborn care, considerable information may need to be transmitted by telephone prior to transport. Almost every child requiring transport needs a well-functioning nasogastric tube that is being frequently aspirated to prevent vomiting and aspiration pneumonia. When lesions such as diaphragmatic hernia are suspected, continuous aspiration of the nasogastric tube may help to prevent further entry of air into the gastrointestinal tract with attendant further compromise of the thoracic space and cardiorespiratory function.

If an intravenous line has not been started, it is usually unnecessary and not worth the time delay and trauma to the baby to have someone attempt it who is not familiar with the techniques. A baby with gastroschisis is an exception to this, for he will lose fluid so rapidly through the exposed bowel surfaces that severe hypovolemia will result if immediate fluid therapy is not provided. Replacement must be with $D_5/RL \pm 5$ percent albumin.[52] Positioning advice may be important in such lesions as esophageal atresia with tracheoesophageal fistula (see Section III).

The most important factor in transport is the availability of a transport service, from either the referring hospital or the neonatal center, which should include a knowledgeable pediatrician familiar with the care problems of the particular surgical anomaly. This may require consultation with the pediatric surgical service prior to transportation.

Before actually embarking, the transporting pediatrician should insure that the baby's temperature is normal, that his airway is clear, that he is well oxygenated, and that he will be able to maintain temperature control and ventilation during the trip. He should provide x-rays, all chart entries, laboratory data, and information about the parents and where they can be reached. A tube of the mother's blood should accompany the baby for subsequent blood cross-matching purposes.

Transport

If all prior arrangements have been handled properly, there should be little to do during the actual transport other than maintaining temperature control and position, if important, and ventilating and oxygenating the baby. Continuous observation for apnea and cyanosis and application of resuscitative techniques when needed complete the pediatrician's responsibilities (Fig. 3). Intubation of an infant en route is hazardous and difficult and should rarely be needed if the problems were properly assessed and treated before embarking. Surface ambulance transport is generally preferable to helicopter transport. The latter is dramatic, but the lack of monitoring of the baby and inability to manipulate the airway make it less beneficial.

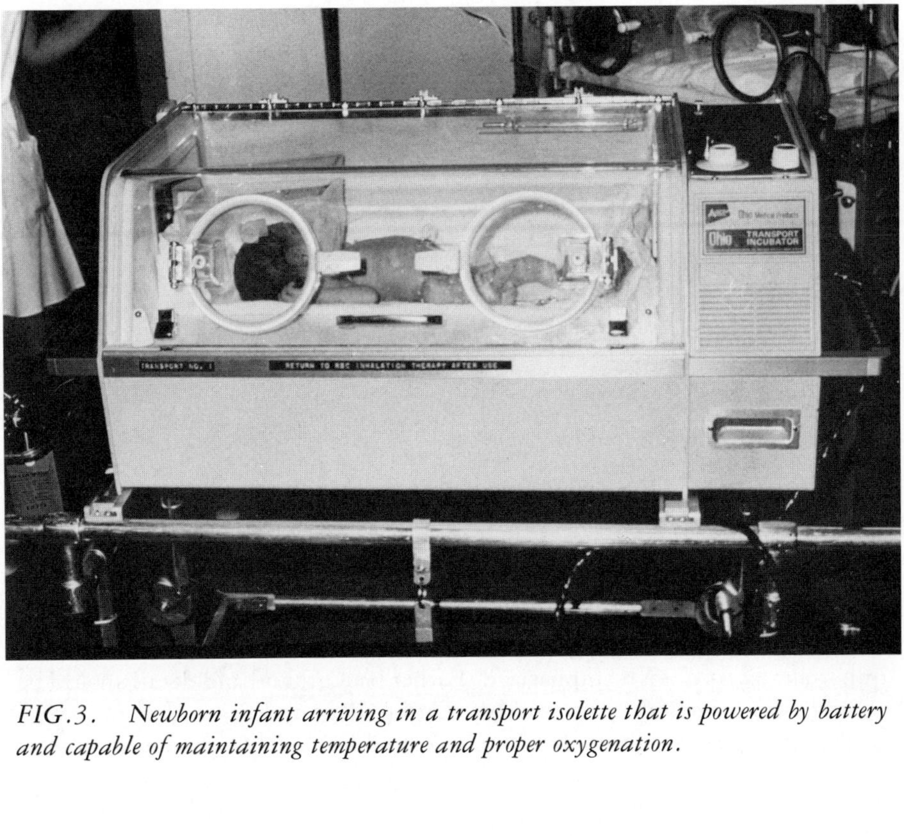

FIG. 3. Newborn infant arriving in a transport isolette that is powered by battery and capable of maintaining temperature and proper oxygenation.

INITIAL CARE OF THE ARRIVING NEONATE

Once the baby has been transported, continued diligence is mandatory to maintain homeostasis and achieve further resuscitation. The following categories of management deserve careful attention:

1. Temperature maintenance—neutral thermal environment
2. Evaluation and support of respiration
   a. Airway management
   b. Oxygenation
   c. Apnea
   d. Ventilatory insufficiency
3. Cardiovascular status
4. Acid–base balance
5. Initial laboratory evaluation
   a. Blood gases—pH
   b. Electrolytes
   c. BUN
   d. Blood glucose
   e. Bilirubin
6. Establishment of venous and arterial cannulas
7. Screening x-ray studies and special studies for diagnosis and treatment
8. Nutritional maintenance
9. Sepsis prevention and treatment
10. Organ system functioning related to newborn physiologic immaturity

Within the scope of this book, these topics, which form the basic outline for a textbook of neonatology, can only be touched on and some of the more important facets of each emphasized. Futher background and detail should be obtained from a suitable text such as that of Klaus and Fanaroff.[53]

The first four categories are closely related and, although certain aspects lend themselves to individual discussion, the maintenance of proper temperature, respiratory sufficiency, pH normality, and cardiovascular perfusion of vital organs must all be considered together for adequate understanding. All must be maintained at normal levels for homeostasis of the infant.

Temperature Maintenance

Newborn infants, particularly premature infants, have inadequate thermal regulatory abilities. Constant diligence is required to keep the baby warm. Cooling leads to increased metabolism, raising oxygen requirements.[18,54,55] Under anesthesia, hypothermia *slows* metabolism and lessens oxygen demand. In the unanesthetized state, however, the patient *increases* his metabolic rate in an attempt to maintain thermal neutrality. This requires a marked increase in oxygen availability at the tissue or cellular level. In addition, as loss of heat continues, the baby begins to vasoconstrict peripherally to protect core temperature. This reduced peripheral circulation leads to anaerobic metabolism with buildup of acid waste products. These are injurious locally and are subsequently released to the general circulation, producing systemic acidosis. Thus, protection from cooling is an essential first step in maintaining circulatory and cardiovascular–respiratory normality.

Generally, exogenous heat sources are required. An isolette is most efficient, but it may be cumbersome for manipulations and procedures. Heating mattresses, overhead heat shields, and raising room temperature are all helpful, but the most important factor is constant vigilance by an aware medical–nursing team (Fig.4).

Particularly with regard to the sick premature infant, simply providing a warm environment may not be adequate. The concept of a neutral thermal environment, whereby sufficient external heat is supplied to allow an infant of given weight and gestational age to maintain normal temperature without any increased metabolic activity, should be thoroughly understood.[54]

From the above discussion it is obvious that at whatever point the knowledgeable neonatal physician enters the picture, he must immediately maximize efforts to obtain and maintain thermal neutrality.

Evaluation and Support of Respiration

While warming measures are being initiated, rapid evaluation of respiratory sufficiency is essential. Although initially observation for general appearance, dyspnea, cyanosis, and airway obstruction may be adequate, early confirmation by arterial blood gas determination is essential. Throughout this evaluation, bear in mind that the Po_2 best indicates oxygenation and Pco_2 represents the state of ventilatory sufficiency.

Most neonatal problems related to pulmonary function are similar to those at any age: airway maintenance, oxygenation, alveolar capillary diffusion, and related acidosis problems. Unique to the neonate are his reduced pulmonary reserve capacity, his sensitivity to hypoxia and acidosis, and the frequency of apneic episodes in premature infants. Further, the small caliber of the infant's tracheobronchial tree leads to much earlier airway obstruction from secretion problems than in the older child or adult.

Finally, the high incidence of hyaline membrane disease, particularly in premature infants with gestational ages of 30 to 36 weeks, makes this serious underlying respiratory insufficiency a frequent accompaniment of many congenital anomalies. It must be remembered that these respiratory deficiencies are the usual inadequacies of the newborn. When anomalies occur which further impair respiratory function, such as diaphragmatic hernia or gastrointestinal obstructions with attendant aspiration pneumonias, these are superimposed on a respiratory system that at best is barely adequate and has minimal margins of safety. Thus, immediate evaluation, rapid and intelligent resuscitative procedures, and considerable skill at ventilatory assistance are essential. (See Chapter 4, Section I, on airway management for further elaboration.)

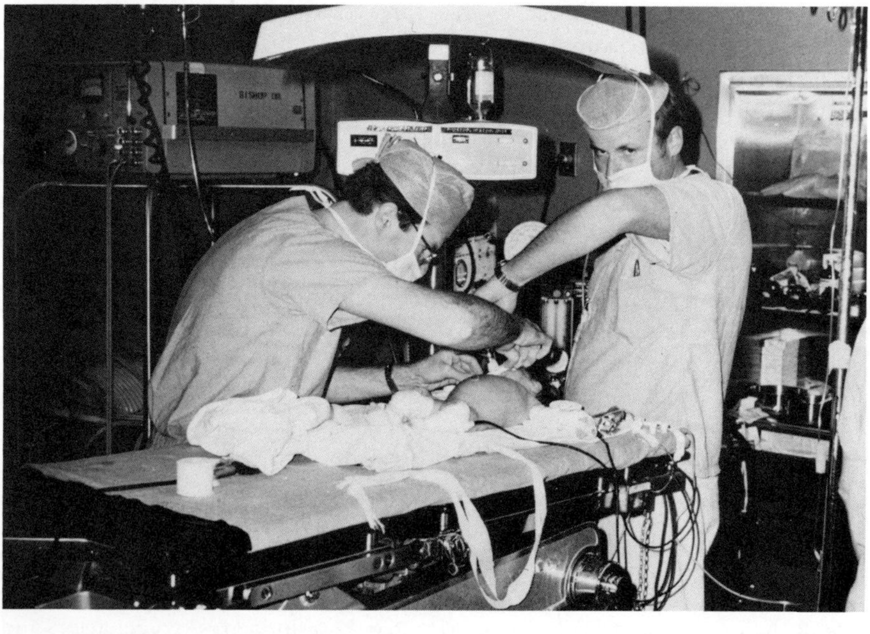

FIG. 4. Anesthesia team preparing infant. Baby lies on a circulating liquid warming mattress under an overhead radiant warmer.

Cardiovascular Status

Although many infants have cardiovascular anomalies that eventually present serious functional problems, only a few very severe cyanosis-producing anomalies cause problems in the newborn period. However, all these infants have an unstable cardiovascular system in that they can easily revert to the fetal pattern. Even though the ductus arteriosus may close functionally within a few minutes after birth,[55] anatomic closure may not come for weeks or months.[56] Any factor such as hypoxia, acidosis, or interstitial pulmonary edema, which increases resistance in the pulmonary vascular circuit, may cause the infant to revert to the fetal state by "shunting" from right to left through the ductus.[55,57–59]

Furthermore, much has been written about the normal newborn's expanded extracellular fluid volume and his ability to tolerate relative dehydration for several days.[11,12] This does not obviate the requirement for careful attention to vascular hypovolemia in the child with abnormal losses such as one with fluid shifts into an obstructed gastrointestinal tract, intraperitoneal losses as a result of peritonitis from perforation, extracapillary losses as a result of membrane injury from sepsis, or even the continuous loss of saliva in a baby with esophageal atresia.

In the presence of reduced vascular volume the infant has the ability to contract to an absolute core circulation, depriving peripheral and mesenteric tissues of oxygen to the point of actual cellular damage with its attendant marked acidosis.[60] Subsequent vasodilatation and loss of capillary integrity may greatly compound fluid losses into the tissues, furthering hypovolemia. This low-flow syndrome is diagramed in Figure 5.

The pulmonary consequences of this state may be marked interstitial edema from capillary damage or from intravascular oncotic deficiency, resulting from protein losses through damaged peripheral capillaries. This edema interferes with oxygen and eventually carbon dioxide transport across the alveolar capillary membranes, worsening hypoxia and acidosis and "recycling" the problem.[23] Thus, proper maintenance of good tissue perfusion through adequate volume replacement and maintenance is essential.

Acid–Base Balance

Proper attention to temperature control, respiratory support, and volume repletion usually results in normal acid–base balance, unless generalized sepsis or some area of tissue necrosis supervenes. However, in the rapidly changing situation of the ill neonate, when assurance of proper homeostasis is mandatory, frequent reevaluation of arterial blood gases and pH is essential. In the first 12 to 24 hours after birth, a mild residual acidosis resulting from the hypoxia and anaerobic metabolism of the delivery process is common.[61] A pH in the range 7.30 to 7.35 is usual. Anything less than this suggests a

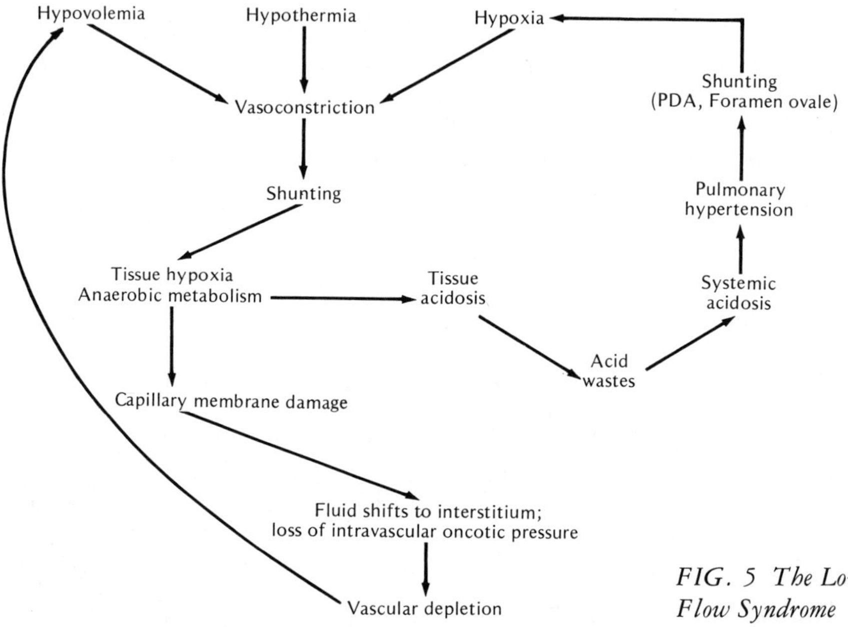

FIG. 5 The Low Flow Syndrome

continuing acidotic load on either a metabolic or hypoxic basis and should be evaluated. By 24 hours of postnatal existence a normal pH is expected.[55]

Initial Laboratory Evaluation

As soon as the child is warm and reasonably stable, the following studies should be obtained:

Determination	**Minimal Blood Required (ml)**
CBC	0.1
Electrolytes	1
BUN/blood glucose	1
Calcium	1
Bilirubin	0.5
Culture	1
Blood gases and pH	0.5
Total	5.1
Optional	
Type and cross-match	3.0
Coombs	
Total	8.1

These are minimum volumes needed by a highly mechanized laboratory using microtechniques. Most of the time, greater volumes are demanded, especially at off-hours by less experienced technicians.

The importance of micromethods in the laboratory and of maximizing information obtainable from a given quantity of blood can be seen by the following table, which lists the blood volumes of representative-weight infants and the corresponding percentages of these volumes represented by this total blood sample. (Newborn blood volume is approximately 8 percent of body weight):[18]

Weight of Infants (g)	Blood Volume (cc)	Blood Volume Drawn (%)
1000	80	10
1500	120	6.67
2000	160	5
2500	200	4
3000	240	3.33

Blood urea nitrogen, calcium, and culture are of importance primarily for establishing baselines. The culture results may subsequently be invaluable. Blood glucose levels are particularly important in the small for gestational age premature infants whose liver glycogen stores and hepatic gluconeogenesis are deficient. Infants of diabetic mothers are likely to be hypoglycemic and dehydrated, and some surgical anomalies, such as omphalocele, may have associated metabolic defects such as the hypoglycemia of the Beckwith syndrome.[62]

A complete discussion of bilirubin metabolism is beyond the scope of this section. The realization that hyperbilirubinemia frequently accompanies major congenital gastrointestinal anomalies, especially atresias of the proximal small intestine, will alert the surgeon to this problem.[63–65] Hyperbilirubinemia is a common physiologic problem of the newborn, is more prevalent in the premature infant, and is usually easily controllable with simple methods if attended to early in its course. The exact levels at which corrective measures are to be instituted should be decided by knowledgeable consultants and therapy guided by them. However, a useful rule of thumb is that, when any baby under the age of 4 days reaches a bilirubin level of 9 mg%, consultation with the neonatologist should be sought and bilirubin determinations should be obtained on a 6-hour schedule.

More serious causes of hyperbilirubinemia can be present in the newborn period including Rh and ABO blood incompatibilities and hemolysis from severe sepsis. These should be ruled out on the initial evaluation. Biliary atresia, neonatal hepatitis, and choledochal cysts almost never present with hyperbilirubinemia in the first few days of life.

Establishment of Venous and Arterial Cannulas

The routine dependence on surgical cutdowns with their attendant vein destruction and permanent scarring should be unnecessary today in any institution that frequently treats newborns. Modern techniques and equipment allow for a wide choice of sites and cannulas that can provide secure, dependable entry sites for monitoring, blood sampling, and fluid and medication administration.

Our preferred method for venous cannulation utilizes a plastic cannula (20 or 22 gauge) passed percutaneously into an antecubital vein or one on the dorsum of the hand.[66] For arterial monitoring or gas determinations we favor an umbilical artery cannula (3½ French) in the umbilical artery.[67] This artery can be transposed to the lower abdomen in the case of omphaloceles or gastroschises or in any situation in which it is preferable to move the line away from the umbilicus.[68]

A reasonable second choice for arterial cannulation is a plastic cannula,* placed either percutaneously or by cutdown into the radial artery at the wrist. Continuous infusions at 2.0 ml/hour of heparinized solutions using a small pump will best maintain patency.[69]

When a cutdown is necessary a useful technique is to pass an umbilical artery catheter (3½ French) centrally from an antecubital entry point. A Castro-y-Juevo cyclodialysis spatula facilitates catheter insertion. Preparation of the entire upper extremity so that it can be elevated above the baby's head while the catheter is being advanced improves the chances for successful central positioning. This central catheter provides a means for both total parenteral alimentation and central venous pressure monitoring and is therefore far more useful than the antiquated saphenous vein ankle cutdown, long the mainstay of infant care. These techniques do require special skills and equipment, and the methodologies are obtainable from the literature. Further details and references are provided in the section on monitoring in Chapter 3, Section I.

Screening X-ray Studies

As discussed in many of the sections on specific lesions, early plain x-rays of the chest and abdomen, including lateral projections, are essential to proper diagnosis and care of most neonatal anomalies. A reiteration of the caution that the newborn's environmental temperature be carefully controlled is important here. Many an infant has deteriorated markedly from prolonged hypothermia during x-ray studies, some to the point of cardiorespiratory arrest! Ideally, screening x-ray evaluations should be obtainable in the newborn unit, obviating the need to transport the newborn to a less optimal environment.

Further studies will depend on the suspected anomaly and the results of screening plain films. The following general points should be recalled:

1. Large and small bowel cannot be differentiated in a child under the age of 2 years on the basis of markings or position except when air is clearly present in the pelvic colon (Fig. 6).

*Argyle Medicut, Sherwood Medical Industries, Inc., St. Louis, Mo.

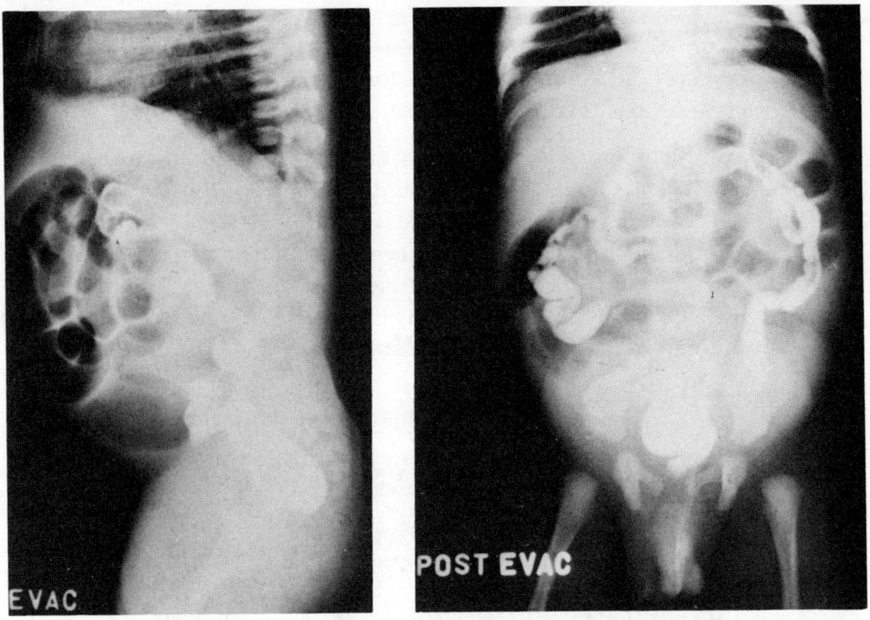

FIG. 6. Contrast enema superimposed on dilated small bowel loops showing "colon-like" pattern of small bowel in the splenic flexure area that could easily be mistaken for colon. The lesion was a distal ileal atresia.

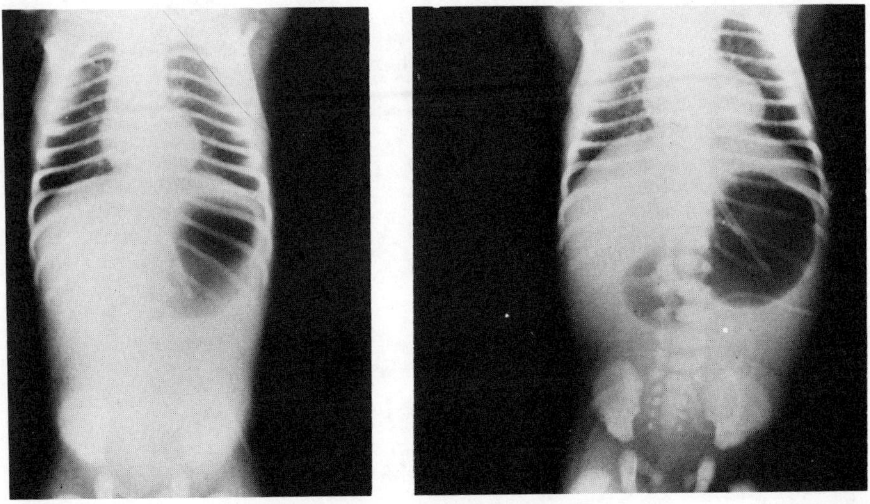

FIG. 7. Plain radiograph of the abdomen in a child with neonatal duodenal obstruction from malrotation showing usefulness of air as an upper intestinal contrast medium.

2. Air is an excellent contrast medium for newborn upper gastrointestinal obstructive lesions (Fig. 7).

3. Water-soluble contrast media are therapeutic when used for evaluation of such entities as meconium ileus and meconium plug.[70,71] However, their high osmolarities produce massive fluid shifts, which may lead to hypovolemic shock.[72] They should never be used without a dependable intravenous line having been established, and immediate fluid replacement with albumin 5 percent in Ringer's lactate should accompany their successful entry into any part of the small intestine.

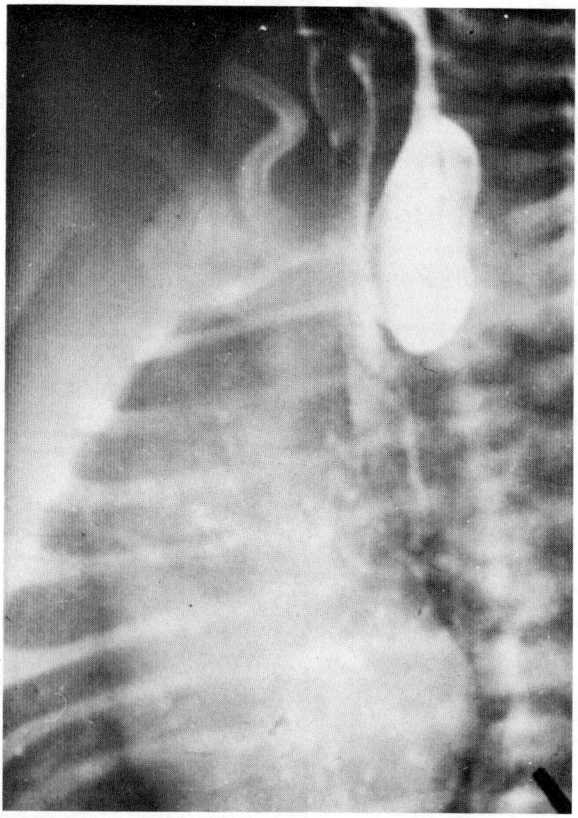

FIG. 8. Aspiration of water-soluble contrast medium into tracheobronchial tree after unnecessary injection of contrast into blind proximal pouch of infant with esophageal atresia.

4. Water-soluble, highly osmolar contrast agents should never be used when the possibility of tracheobronchial aspiration is present as in esophageal atresia or upper gastrointestinal obstruction, for their effect on the ciliated respiratory epithelium is devasting (Fig. 8).

Nutritional Maintenance

Once the initial evaluation outlined above is completed, an estimate of the time span likely to pass before normal gastrointestinal function is possible should be made. Except for the premature infant, with an increased tendency toward hypoglycemia, most newborns can tolerate several days of low caloric levels as long as good fluid and electrolyte management and 5 percent dextrose are maintained. When more than six or seven days without progress to normal gastrointestinal alimentation are anticipated, the baby will definitely benefit from early establishment of intravenous central alimentation.

Prevention and Treatment of Sepsis

Sepsis is one of the major causes of death in infants with anomalies requiring surgical management. The diagnosis of sepsis in early infancy can be quite difficult, as the signs and symptoms are often minimal. Unlike older children and adults, the septic infant not only fails to show fever, but is more likely to show a depression in temperature. The baby's color and general appearance may be poor, representing generalized decrease in tissue/organ perfusion. Urine output may remain adequate until very late stages, however. Vomiting may be an early sign, as an ileus develops secondary to the sepsis. The baby also may be less active than previously. Bradycardia and apnea are common, especially in small premature infants.

The newborn has an immature immune defense mechanism and little or no antigenic experience. He is unable to call forth a rapid and effective defense against bacteria and may therefore be easily overwhelmed by infectious challenges that would be contained and localized by an older child. The baby is born with some immunoglobulin G, which is passed transplacentally. Immunoglobulins M and A are essentially absent. In fact, the presence of IgM in a newborn suggests in utero infection.[73] In addition to immunoglobulin deficiency the newborn's leukocytes lack a complement factor important for opsonization and phagocytosis. Therefore, both major defense mechanisms, cellular and humoral immunity, are immature and incompetent.

In view of this immune deficiency, prophylactic antibiotic coverage seems warranted, especially for any procedure involving contamination of any kind. We have generally used preoperative antibiotics in most newborns, but there is not total agreement with this position.

Gram-negative organisms are the usual invaders, especially if antibiotic coverage has been provided prophylactically or therapeutically for other infections. Disseminated intravascular coagulopathy (DIC) may follow shortly after the onset of sepsis. Once the full-blown picture of DIC is present, the chances of reversing the sepsis and saving the baby are low. Thus, early recognition of sepsis and appropriate antibiotic, fluid, and blood or plasma therapy are most important.

The value of the platelet count for monitoring the state of the clotting mechanism and detecting early sepsis cannot be overemphasized. All surgical neonates and infants should have regular determinations of platelets, and, if a significant fall occurs, rapid evaluation, blood cultures, and appropriate therapy should be instituted. An antibiotic with good coverage for resistant gram-negative organisms such as *Klebsiella* and *Pseudomonas* should be included in the therapeutic regimen. Gentamycin is an excellent choice.

Delay in initiating therapy must not be tolerated. The rapidity of the destructive course of gram-negative sepsis does not allow time to await culture results or formal clotting factor evaluations. Blood should be drawn for these determinations, however, to confirm the diagnosis and guide subsequent therapy.

When severe generalized sepsis occurs, the need for fluid to maintain vascular volume is increased. At the same time, pulmonary and cardiovascular decompensation may accompany the severe toxic state, as the lungs and heart share in the generalized cellular injury. Ventilatory assistance may be required, and cardiac decompensation may require digitalization to enable the toxic myocardium to handle the circulatory needs in the acute septic phase. One should not hesitate to digitalize such a baby even though his heart is otherwise normal. Without the help of the digitalis, the heart in this toxic phase may not be able to handle the fluid loads needed to maintain vascular volume and tissue/organ perfusion. This leads to the serious and complex state of a child in both congestive failure and hypovolemic shock simultaneously. Dopamine* is probably a better first choice here, as it will improve both myocardial function and renal perfusion without the attendant risk of arrhythmias that accompanies the use of digitalis.

Recently the use of steroids in septic and shock states has had much investigation. They supposedly maintain the integrity of the lysosomal membranes, preventing the release of destructive enzymes therefrom. This has not been consistently demonstrable.[74] Their efficacy in maintaining the integrity of other membranes, such as pulmonary capillary walls, is still being studied.

Finally, the successful reversal of disseminated intravascular coagulopathy by totally exchanging the child's blood has now been accomplished frequently enough to establish this as a most efficacious treatment.[30] Multiple such exchanges may be required to maintain improvement and overcome the clotting disturbance. We have utilized as many as 26 exchanges with eventual survival of a healthy infant.

*Intropin, Arnar-Stone Laboratories, Inc., Mount Prospect, Ill.

Organ System Functioning Related to Newborn Physiologic Immaturity

Only the briefest outline is possible here. Some of this area has already been covered above.

1. Neurologic: Immature reflexes, premature tendency to apnea, need for essential fatty acids during long-term parenteral alimentation to enable myelinization of the central nervous system to proceed normally.

2. Endocrine: No significant abnormality; functions quite well.

3. Cardiovascular: Fetal circulation, tendency to severe constriction to core circulation in response to cold, hypovolemia, hypoxia, and acidosis, producing low-flow syndrome.

4. Respiratory: Apnea, high incidence of hyaline membrane disease, susceptibility to intrapulmonary shunting and hypertension with restoration of fetal circulatory pattern through ductus arteriosus or foramen ovale bypassing the lung.

5. Hepatic: Immature enzyme systems, leading to slow degradation of metabolic breakdown products and some drugs.

6. Gastrointestinal: Occasional intolerances such as disaccharidase deficiency and malabsorption-type syndromes.

7. Urinary: Deficiencies much overstated, but kidney's ability to concentrate or dilute at extremes less developed than in older child or adult. Specifically, will waste sodium in the face of sodium depletion in the extracellular fluid. Will sort things out quite well, however, if adequate fluid and electrolytes are provided.

CHAPTER 3

MODERN MONITORING AND SUPPORT TECHNIQUES FOR INFANTS

INTRAVENOUS THERAPY

PURPOSE

Intravenous therapy is used to maintain fluids and electrolytes, to supply essential nutrients, minerals, and vitamins, and to administer drugs.

AVAILABLE SITES

As in adults, any visible or palpable vein is appropriate. The veins of the antecubital fossa, dorsum of the hand, and ventral surface of the wrist are most useful, as are those of the scalp. Femoral cannulations should be avoided except in extreme emergencies, as the risk of sepsis is increased with their use.

METHODS

Butterfly Needles

Butterfly needles are useful for short-term fluid therapy and blood drawing. Their disadvantages are that they are unstable and undependable because of the ease of the needle cutting through the vein and extravasating fluid.

Plastic Cannulas

Plastic cannulas are placed percutaneously by means of an inner metal needle stylet, which is then removed. A model with one-piece tapered-hub construction of clear plastic is our preference.* The details of its placement are described in the following sections.[66]†

EQUIPMENT

1. A 20-gauge percutaneous venous cannula constructed as a tapered plastic sheath surrounding a removable metal stylet with syringe attached. This is referred to subsequently as the percutaneous venous cannula.
2. An 18-gauge needle.
3. A padded armboard splint.
4. Antiseptic solution for preparation of the skin.
5. Standard intravenous fluid administration set with pediatric control chamber.
6. A short segment of extension tubing or "T-connection" for the intravenous tubing.
7. Usual tourniquet, tape, and fluids for intravenous therapy.

VENIPUNCTURE TECHNIQUE

Because success with this technique requires meticulous attention to seemingly obvious points, discussion of details and equipment used is essential.

The antecubital veins of the forearm are preferred, but the veins on the dorsum of the hands or ventral surface of the wrist are used frequently, especially in smaller infants. Antiseptic solution is used on both the patient and the physician's palpating finger. The site must then be dried with sterile gauze to allow traction during insertion. A soft, padded armboard approximately 10 × 20 cm is used. Rolled gauze padding is used behind the elbow to hyperextend the antecubital fossa. Waterproof tape is essential. The armboard is then taped to the table or mattress for complete immobilization of the extremity. The baby is placed on the table so that, with the arm extended, there is still room for the physician to stabilize his hand on the table surface. A medium-sized rubber band is an ideal tourniquet (Fig.9).

Many products for percutaneous venous cannulation are available on the market, but the one chosen must have the following features:

1. An inner metal needle as stylet with a clear chamber in the hub for early detection of aspirated blood.

2. An outer plastic cannula that is gently tapered at the distal end to permit easy insertion into tiny veins.

*Argyle Medicut, Sherwood Medical Industries, Inc., St. Louis, Mo.

†This material originally appeared in Pediatrics 48:896, 1971, and is presented here with the kind permission of the American Academy of Pediatrics.[66]

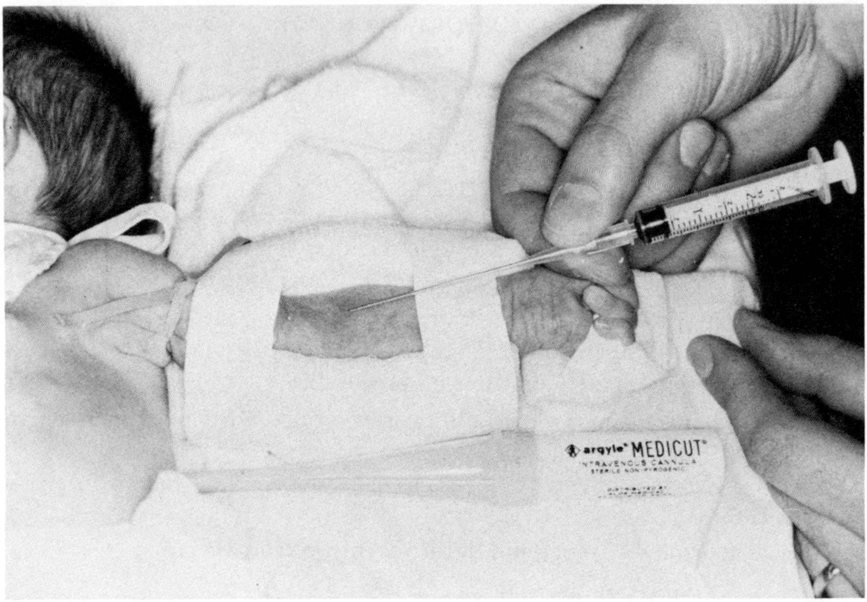

FIG.9. The baby's arm is immobilized preparatory to insertion of plastic intravenous cannula. A rubber band tourniquet is in place.

3. A tapered hub end that is an integral part of the cannula. This eliminates the connection of catheter to metal hub with its risk of disconnection and embolism.

4. An attached syringe with an airtight connection to the stylet hub.

A standard 18-gauge needle is used to puncture the skin approximately 1 cm from the proposed site of venipuncture and in line with the direction of the vein. The percutaneous venous cannula is then inserted, *bevel down*, through the skin puncture site and advanced slowly toward the vein. Negative pressure is applied to the barrel of the syringe, and the clear chamber is observed for the first sign of blood aspiration as the cannula is advanced. The importance of inserting the needle with the bevel down is shown in Figure 10. In a small vein the point of a needle inserted with the bevel up passes through the back wall of the vessel before the lumen of the needle reaches the lumen of the vein. Thus, by the time the blood is aspirated into the syringe and success of the venipuncture is recognized, the needle has passed through both walls of the vein. When the needle is inserted bevel down, the point advances into the lumen of the vein in line with the lumen of the needle. Therefore, blood aspiration is apparent in the hub chamber before the back wall is pierced, and the cannula can then be advanced into the lumen of the vein.

The cannula must be advanced slowly in fractions of a millimeter. The index finger of the opposite hand is used to palpate the relationship between the needle point and the vein. The venipuncture is performed directly into the upper surface of the vein.

Once successful entry is confirmed by the return of blood into the viewing chamber of the needle hub, approximately 1 ml of blood is withdrawn into the syringe. The hand holding the syringe is carefully braced against the table top and the thumb of that hand used to reinject the blood into the vessel, thus distending it. Simultaneously, the hand advances the whole syringe, needle, and plastic catheter as a unit forward a few millimeters into the lumen of the vein. This allows the plastic catheter with its slight "lip" to puncture the vein wall and enter the lumen while the needle tip is advancing easily into the blood-distended lumen ahead of it (Fig. 11). Usually a distinct "pop" can be felt as the catheter traverses the vein wall. If this step is omitted

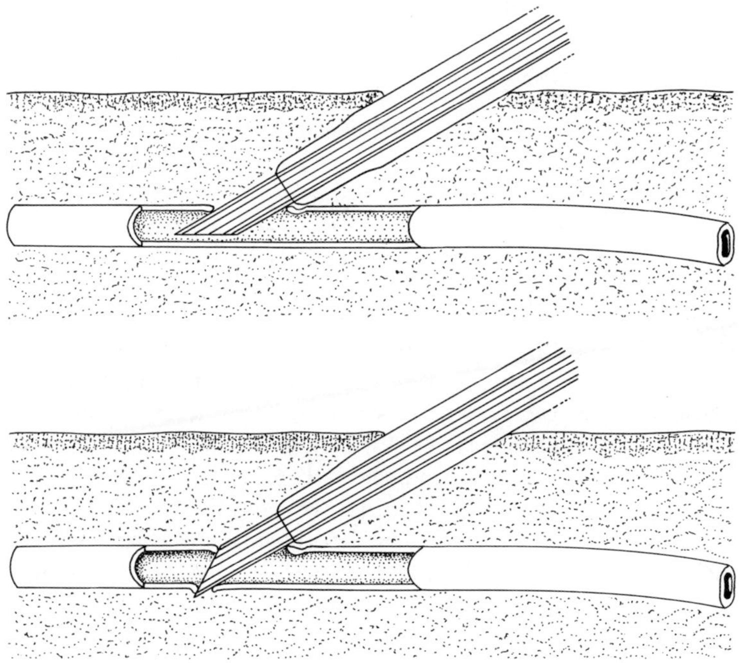

FIG. 10. Above: With the needle point inserted bevel down, *the lumen of the needle enters the midlumen of the tiny vein. Below: When the venipuncture is performed* bevel up, *the needle point pierces the deep wall of the vessel before blood return is apparent. (From Filston and Johnson: Pediatrics 48:896, 1971; © American Academy of Pediatrics, Inc., 1971)*

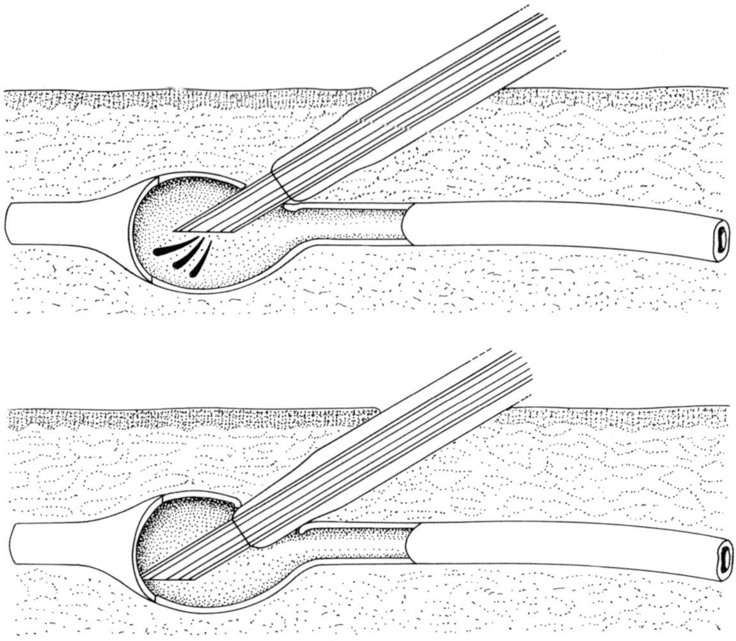

FIG.11. Above: Reinjection of the aspirated blood expands the vessel, leaving room for further advancement of the needle. Below: The plastic catheter lip can then enter the lumen of the vessel without the needle perforating the deep wall. (From Filston and Johnson: Pediatrics 48:896, 1971; © American Academy of Pediatrics, Inc., 1971)

and the catheter is merely pushed forward after the needle enters the vein, the edge of the catheter will push the vein wall off the end of the needle, and the procedure will fail. Once the plastic catheter has entered the vessel lumen, the inner needle stylet can be withdrawn and the catheter advanced inward until the flare of the hub binds at the skin puncture site. When the procedure is successful, a free flow of blood from the catheter hub is noted after removal of the stylet. If no such flow is present, either the catheter never entered the lumen or the entire cannula has traversed both walls and the vessel has been transfixed by the catheter. If the latter is the case, a successful cannulation can usually be salvaged by slowly withdrawing the plastic catheter (without reinserting the stylet) until a free flow of blood is noted. Rotation and advancement of the catheter will then place it into the lumen properly. Free flow of blood will persist. If the catheter has not entered the lumen at all, free blood flow may be noted when its tip is opposite the needle puncture site, but after rotation and readvancement the blood flow will again cease.

Antibiotic ointment is used to cover the puncture site on the skin and is covered with a small Band-aid dressing. If the catheter is allowed any room to slide back and forth, it will soon leak. The arm is therefore coated with

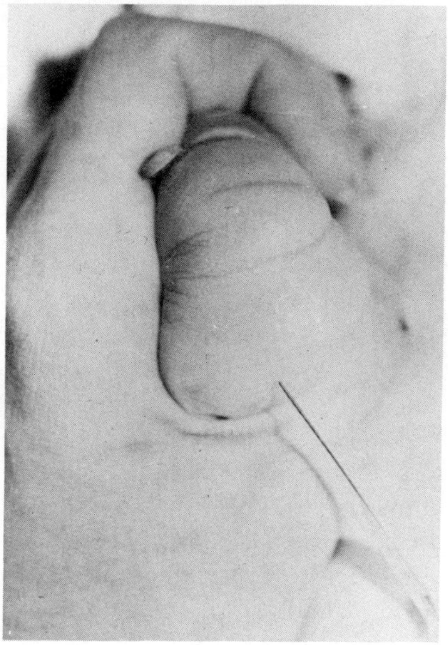

FIG.12. Correct immobilization of infant's wrist and hand for insertion of cannula into dorsal hand veins.

tincture of benzoin solution, and a long strip of waterproof tape is used to secure the catheter. Additional strips of tape are then used to further anchor the catheter. Immobilization is accomplished by readjusting the padded armboard splint. The child must not be allowed to flex at the elbow, as this will crimp or break the plastic catheter. Rolls of 4 × 4 gauze sponges are placed along each side of the arm bridging the elbow. The armboard splint is then taped in place. To facilitate daily solution and tubing changes, a T-Connector* is inserted into the cannula and the IV line is then connected into this. In this manner, the IV bottle, tubing, and administration set can be changed daily without disturbing the catheter. If the IV tubing is connected directly into the catheter, the motion of changing the tubing connection will enlarge the venipuncture and cause leakage. It is mandatory to inspect the cannula daily to be certain that it is still functioning properly and phlebitis is not developing. It is usually unnecessary to untape the cannula completely to make this inspection.

Frequently, in tiny infants, the vessels on the dorsum of the hand or ventral surface of the wrist are more easily cannulated. In these cases, the arm is not attached to a board until successful cannulation is accomplished. The infant's hand is held by the physician in such a way as to put maximum stretch on the vein. For the dorsum of the hand, this requires complete flexion of the infant's wrist such that the ventral surfaces of the hand and fingers appose the ventral forearm. The physician must not place his hand between the infant's forearm and ventral hand surface, as this will leave the veins too lax (Fig. 12).

*T-Connector, Abbott Laboratories, Chicago, Ill.

Incisional Cutdowns for Venous Cannulation

With a little practice and experience percutaneous cannulation becomes so simple that incisional cutdown is rarely necessary. When it is, central placement of a long plastic cannula should be considered because it offers the added advantages over peripheral short catheters of longevity, monitoring availability (central venous pressure), and concentrated nutritional support (see section on central venous pressure monitoring, p. 56).

Occasionally, peripheral cutdown cannulation is still required. When it is, only the smallest nick need be made on the skin overlying the vein. A mosquito hemostat is used to elevate the vein into the wound. A ligature is looped around the vein for traction but is not tied. The same type of plastic cannula–needle stylet system is then used to puncture the vein under direct vision without an incision. The plastic cannula is advanced fully, the ligature removed, and the catheter taped in place in the same fashion as when placed percutaneously. In this way a larger-sized catheter can usually be used because the vein remains distended with blood. In addition, the vein is not ligated and is therefore frequently preserved for subsequent use.

ARTERIAL BLOOD GAS AND pH MONITORING

INTRODUCTION

Purpose

The purpose is to monitor the respiratory function and acid–base balance of the infant in order to provide needed ventilatory support and buffering therapy to sustain homeostasis.

Principles

Arterial blood gases and pH provide the surest measurement of the infant's homeostasis. The PO_2 primarily indicates the ability of oxygen to diffuse through the alveolar capillary membranes. Deficiencies are corrected by increasing inspired oxygen or by increasing the pressure at which the gases are delivered during the cycle. The latter is achieved by either continuous positive airway pressure (CPAP) or positive end expiratory pressure (PEEP). The effects of the two methods are essentially similar, the major difference being that CPAP is usually used with either nasal prongs or an endotracheal tube without a respirator, whereas PEEP is the usual method of providing increased pressure when a respirator is in use (see the section on respiratory management, pp. 63–75).

Whenever oxygen concentrations above normal air are used or when oxygen is delivered at increased mean pressure (CPAP or PEEP), vigilant Po_2 monitoring is mandatory to insure that Po_2 is not over 100 mm Hg. Levels above 100 in newborns, particularly premature infants, may lead to retrolental fibroplasia (RLF) and leave the baby blind.[75] Even short periods of minimal elevation can produce this in a premature infant. Remember that the development of RLF is dependent on Po_2, not on inspired oxygen concentration. This means that RLF can develop when inspired O_2 is only 25 or 30 mm Hg or when only 3 to 5 cm of PEEP or CPAP are being used. The implications of this for the anesthesiologist dealing with infants should be apparent. Intraoperative monitoring is essential when even moderately long anesthesias at increased inspired oxygen levels are contemplated in premature infants.

The Pco_2, on the other hand, is a measure of ventilatory adequacy, that is, the ability to move air into and out of the alveolus, because CO_2 will continue to diffuse long after severe O_2 block occurs. Thus, when CO_2 is being retained in the blood, this is either a compensation for metabolic alkalosis, or a respiratory acidosis due to ventilatory insufficiency. When Pco_2 levels approach 60 mm Hg, mechanical ventilation should be instituted.

Monitoring of pH is essential to maintain homeostasis. However, pH alone will not give the etiology of acidosis or alkalosis. Bicarbonate and Pco_2 levels must be obtained to differentiate respiratory from metabolic etiologies. The two most common causes of acidosis in infants are ventilatory insufficiency (respiratory acidosis) and ischemic tissue damage due to hypoxia hypovolemia or hypothermia (metabolic acidosis).

TECHNIQUES

Umbilical Artery Cannulation[67]

The umbilical artery is the most common site used. It is readily available in most instances, and cannulation is reasonably simple to perform, as follows:

1. The cord and abdomen are prepared with antiseptic solution.
2. The stump is amputated close to the skin.
3. A heavy ligature or umbilical tape (0.25-inch twill tape) is loosely tied around the base of the cord.
4. The umbilical arteries are identified. One is chosen for cannulation, and its lumen is gently probed and dilated to the diameter of the chosen catheter (3½ or 5 French).
5. The catheter is inserted and passed with firm pressure until blood returns. It is then advanced 1 cm and appropriately fixed in position with suture ligatures and tape.

6. A continuous infusion of solution heparinized with 1 unit heparin per milliliter will maintain patency.

7. The catheter's position should be checked by x-ray. It should be near the bifurcation of the aorta. It should not lie adjacent to the renal or mesenteric ostia.

8. If evidence of peripheral embolization occurs, the catheter should be discontinued. However, vascular insufficiency of the extremities is more often due to the generalized low-flow state of the seriously ill neonate than to thrombosis or embolization related to the presence of the catheter. The use of the term "catheter toes" and "catheter feet" implies an iatrogenic liability that may be unfounded.[76]

Transposition of the Umbilical Artery

This procedure retains the availability of the umbilical vessels when the umbilicus is involved in the surgical field as in omphalocele and gastroschisis. It also has the advantage of removing the vessels from the degenerating umbilical area with its attendant risk of infection. It may therefore have applicability for many intra-abdominal lesions. The technique is simple and has been described elsewhere.[68] (Fig. 13).

Radial Artery Cannulation

This procedure is technically more difficult than umbilical cannulation but is still readily learned. Preferably, the artery is cannulated percutaneously in a fashion similar to percutaneous venous cannulation except that reinjection of aspirated blood is not necessary. The arm is positioned as in step 1 below. When percutaneous cannulation is unsuccessful, the same vessel can be used for open placement.

TECHNIQUE: INCISIONAL RADIAL ARTERY CANNULATION

1. The baby's hand is taped to an 8 × 15 cm padded armboard with the wrist hyperextended over a gauze roll. This places the radial artery on stretch. The arm is further taped to the board proximally with padded gauze rolls on either side. The skin is prepared with antiseptic solution.

2. The radial pulse is palpated and a small 0.5-cm skin incision is made transversely just proximal to the ventral wrist skin creases.

3. The incision is deepened into the subcutaneous tissue with a small clamp (not with the scalpel).

4. A curved mosquito hemostat is used to dissect free and elevate the artery. If the clamp is used to dissect deeply into the tissue at one corner of the wound and then curved back up to the other corner, the artery should be in the tissue that is elevated.

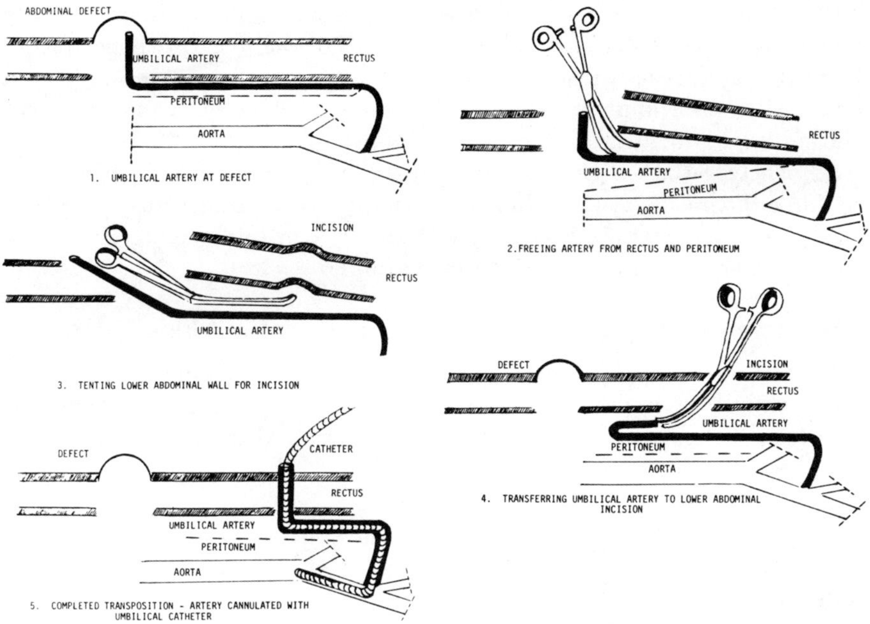

FIG. 13. Schematic representation of technique of transposition of the umbilical artery. (From Filston and Izant: J Pediatr Surg 10:225, 1975)

5. An untied ligature is looped selectively about the artery for traction purposes.

6. Under direct vision a 22-gauge plastic cannula with inner metal needle stylet* is advanced *bevel down* into the artery until the plastic cannula is clearly within the vessel lumen. The stylet is then removed and the cannula advanced to the tapered hub.

7. The ligature is removed. Usually the incision can be kept small enough that the hub of the cannula fills it and no closing suture is needed. If larger than the hub, the incision should be sutured.

8. Tape is used to secure the cannula as described in the section on percutaneous venous cannulation. A T-connector† and three-way stopcock are attached to the hub of the cannula, and continuous heparinized infusion is used to maintain patency of the vessel.

9. No drugs should be administered at this site.

*Argyle Medicut Cannula, Sherwood Medical Industries, Inc., St. Louis, Mo.
†T-connector, Abbott Laboratories, Chicago, Ill.

10. Flush infusions after samples are withdrawn should be injected slowly to avoid arteriolar spasm and ischemic necrosis of the forearm tissues proximal to the cannulation site.

11. All connections must be taped securely to avoid accidental disjunction and exsanguinating hemorrhage.

12. These catheters should not be used in an unattended patient and should be discontinued when blood gas monitoring or direct blood pressure readings are no longer needed. They should not be maintained merely as convenient sites for obtaining routine blood samples.

Temporal Artery Cannulation for Blood Gas Monitoring

The temporal artery is another readily available vessel for monitoring. It is easily cannulated if attention is directed to a few details. Gauderer and Holgersen[77] and more recently Prian[78] have described the technique.

PERCUTANEOUS PLACEMENT OF A SUBCLAVIAN CATHETER FOR CENTRAL VENOUS PRESSURE MONITORING AND TOTAL PARENTERAL NUTRITION

PURPOSE

The purpose is to provide continuous access to the central venous system for central pressure monitoring and full nutritional support.

DISCUSSION

Most infants have such an appropriate urinary response to restored vascular volume that urine output monitoring alone is sufficient to guide fluid therapy. In those infants in whom acidosis, ischemic injury, or sepsis complicate the management of the surgical anomaly, however, myocardial insufficiency, inappropriate antidiuretic hormone secretion, or renal tubular necrosis may make total dependence on urinary output hazardous. In these infants CVP monitoring provides a fail-safe guide to urinary output monitoring and prevents excess fluid overload.[79,80]

TECHNIQUE

Central venous cannulation can be achieved safely by incisional "cutdown" of the basilic vein in the antecubital fossa or by incision over the jugular veins in the neck. The latter technique is the accepted standard procedure for placing TPN catheters in infants.[40] Its disadvantage is that it is tedious to perform, and, unless the deep jugular vein is used, central placement is not always achieved. The same is true of the antecubital route. Also, once used the vein is wasted.

Groff and Ahmed[41] and Morgan and Harkens[42] independently have reported sizable experiences with percutaneous subclavian cannulations. Because of the risks attendant on placement of a subclavicular needle in a tiny baby, we long hesitated to advocate this technique. The recent availability of a system utilizing a plastic cannula placed into the vein with a needle stylet and then allowing the manipulations for central placement of the following long catheter to be performed with only the plastic cannula* in the vein have enabled us to use this technique in well over a hundred infants ranging in size down to 680 g without a complication (Fig. 14).

The physician utilizing this technique must have the following capabilities: (a) extensive experience in placing subclavian catheters in older children and adults; (b) excellent facility in the use of percutaneous peripheral plastic catheters in infants. The procedure, which must be seen as useful but potentially hazardous, is as follows:

1. The cannulation is invariably performed in the operating room with the baby monitored carefully but not anesthetized.

2. The extremities are wrapped and secured to the table with the arms pulled down toward the feet on each side. The table is placed in enough Trendelenberg position (usually all the way) so that the infant himself is definitely head below heels. This helps to fill the veins and prevent air embolism.

3. A small towel serves as a roll beneath the baby's shoulders to allow hyperextension of the neck. The face should point straight forward.

4. An x-ray cassette is placed beneath the warming mattress positioned beneath the neck and chest.

5. A whiskey-sugar nipple will quiet the baby.

6. An overhead radiant heater is used to maintain the infant's temperature.

7. The skin of the neck and chest are prepared with antiseptic solution† and the field draped with towels.

8. One milliliter of 1 percent lidocaine is infiltrated into the skin beneath the clavicle at the chosen puncture site. This site should be at the midpoint of the clavicle.

9. A puncture is made in the skin with a needle larger than the central catheter system.

*Argyle Intramedicut Catheter, Sherwood Medical Industries, St. Louis, Mo.
†Betadine Solution, Purdue Frederick Co., Norwalk, Conn.

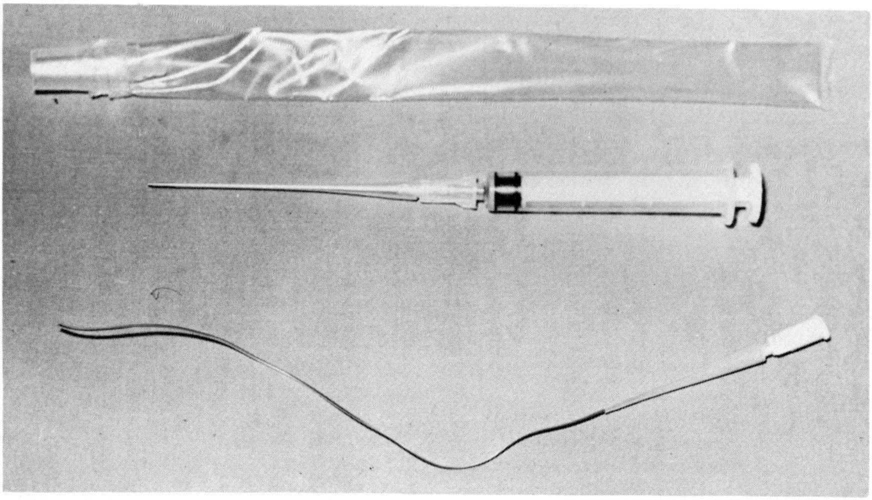

FIG. 14. Equipment for percutaneous placement of a central venous line by the subclavian route. The sterile covering sheath for the catheter makes a handy guide to measure the length of catheter in the baby.

10. The cannula with needle stylet and syringe are flushed with heparinized saline as is the longer following catheter.

11. The cannula is passed just beneath the clavicle, aiming about 1 cm above the sternal notch in a line that approximates the deltopectoral groove. Slight suction is applied to the needle by aspirating the syringe (Fig. 15).

12. The cardinal rule is never to change direction of the needle once it is beneath the clavicle, as this motion would result in a laceration of any structure inadvertently punctured with the needle.[41]

13. If blood returns in the needle, aspirate 0.5 ml or more, reinject it forcefully, and advance the needle with the cannula a few millimeters further into the vessel.

14. If blood fails to return after the needle has been advanced an adequate distance, remove the needle stylet and then slowly back the plastic cannula out.

15. Once satisfactory blood flow is achieved from the cannula, aim it transversely by elevating its proximal end toward the baby's head (do not back it out and dislodge it from the vein). A slight bend should be placed in the long catheter to facilitate its turning downward into the superior vena cava. Pass the catheter into the plastic cannula with the curve pointing caudad relative to the infant and advance it an appropriate distance into the vena cava.

16. Attach the syringe filled with heparinized solution to the catheter, insure that blood can be freely aspirated, infuse some heparinized solution, and prepare for x-ray. Inject 1 ml of intravenous contrast material into the catheter just prior to x-ray to insure against extravascular placement. Do not remove the cannula from the vein until x-ray confirms proper placement of the catheter (Fig. 16).

17. Adjust the positon of the catheter based upon the x-ray findings, back the cannula out of the vein and back to wedge against the catheter hub, and secure the catheter with sutures and tape.

18. Antibiotic ointment and a sterile dressing should be applied to the puncture site.

The catheter is now ready for central venous pressure monitoring or total parenteral nutrition.

When a catheter that has been used for CVP monitoring is later to be used for TPN, all solutions and tubing down to the catheter are changed, and the CVP monitor attachments and stopcocks are removed. The dressing at the puncture site is changed and new antibiotic ointment applied. A blood culture is obtained through the catheter prior to attaching the new tubing. A filter is placed in the line. The line is maintained with heparinized stock solutions. If the blood culture shows no growth after 48 hours, TPN solution is administered through the line.

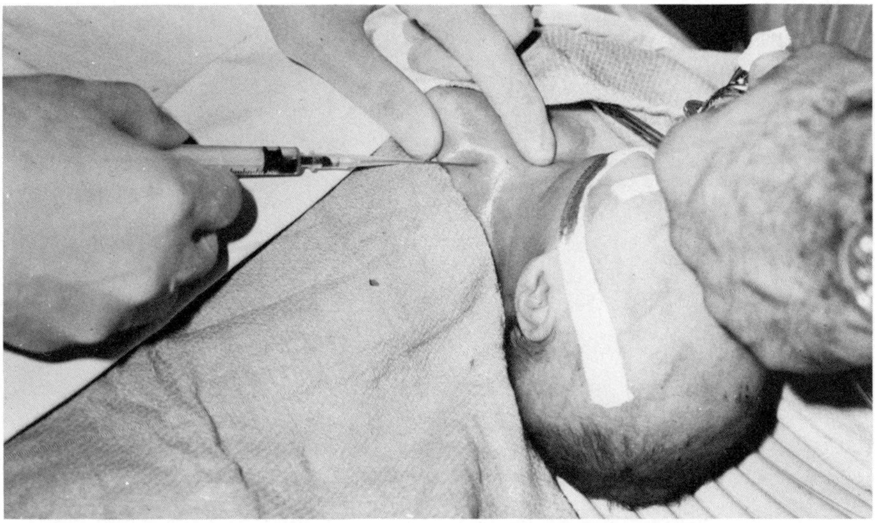

FIG. 15. Infant in position for percutaneous insertion of central catheter. General anesthesia pictured here is not needed unless, as in this case, the cannulation is performed concomitantly with major surgery.

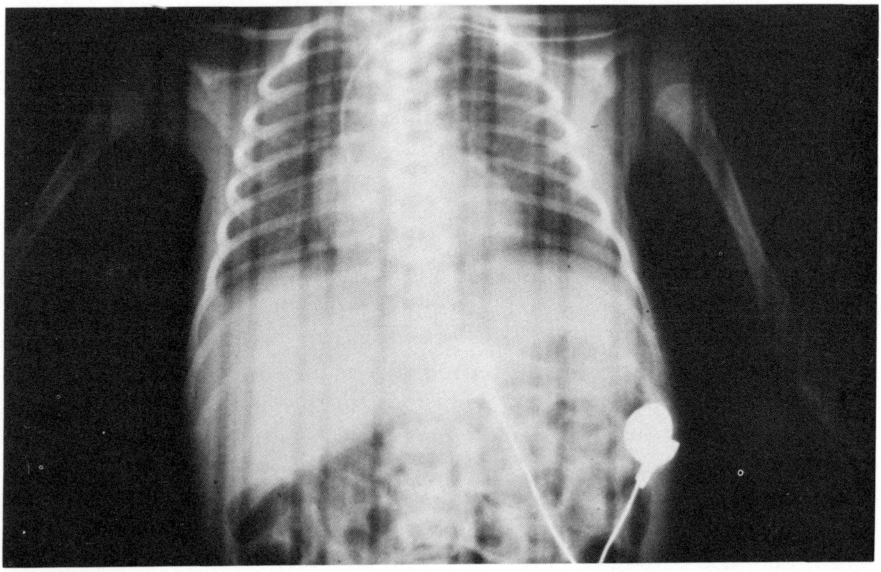

FIG. 16. Chest radiograph showing central catheter properly positioned in superior vena cava from left subclavian.

The greatest advantage of this approach, in addition to its simplicity, is that when prolonged TPN is required the lines can readily be alternated from side to side and the veins recannulated numerous times.

MONITORING VITAL SIGNS IN NEWBORN INFANTS

BLOOD PRESSURE

When an aterial line is in place for arterial blood gas monitoring, it can be used simultaneously for direct readout blood pressure monitoring using a transducer incorporating a continuously flushing system. One such has been described by Johnson and Ito.[69] If an arterial line is not available, a system utilizing the Doppler ultrasound technique* will provide dependable data.

*Roche Arteriosonde, Roche Medical Electronics Division, Hoffman LaRoche, Inc., Cranbury, N.J.

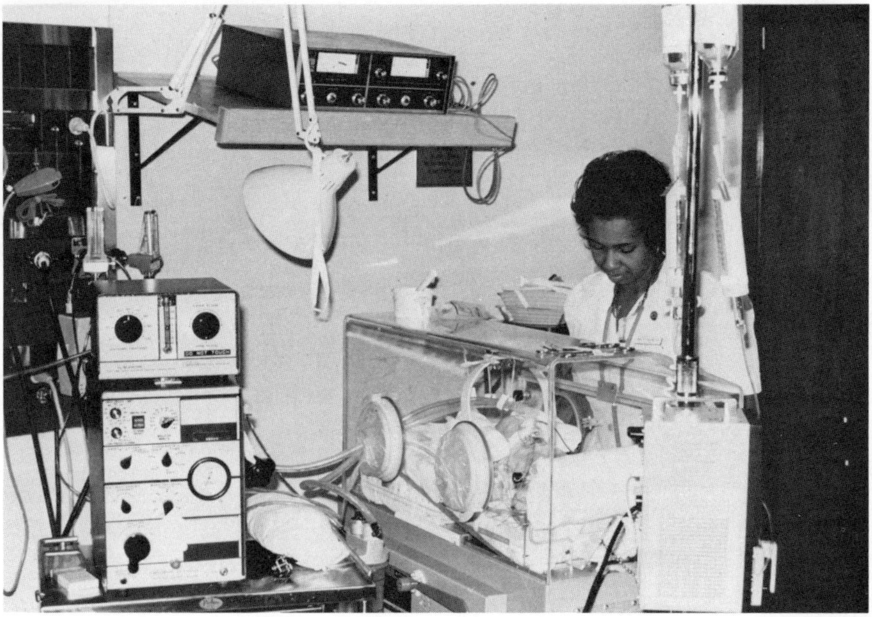

FIG. 17. Major respiratory support and multiple monitoring modalities in a seriously ill postoperative neonate.

RESPIRATIONS

The important entity to monitor is rate, ie, apnea. Various "blanket" mattresses and encircling chest bands are available to electronically monitor respiratory rate in infants and audibly warn of apnea.

HEART RATE, RHYTHM, AND ELECTROCARDIOGRAM

Sophisticated instruments can provide anything from rate monitoring with bradycardia warning to "memory" electrocardiogram recording and instant recall. The most important monitor for the newborn is rate with bradycardia warnings, as this will result from any hypoxic or septic insult (Fig. 17).

TEMPERATURE

Continuous temperature monitoring via skin thermocouples helps to insure the proper environmental temperature. When overhead warmers are used, they should be capable of automatic thermister response to changes in the baby's temperature.

CHAPTER 4

INFANT AIRWAY MANAGEMENT AND VENTILATORY SUPPORT

INTRODUCTION

Perhaps more than any other single aspect of care, the management of the infant's airway and support of his ventilation are the final pathway leading to survival or demise. The tremendous strides that have been achieved with the premature infant in sustaining adequate oxygenation through a wide range of respiratory embarrassments form the basis for the rather sophisticated approaches now being commonly utilized in neonatal centers. The pediatric surgical patient faces many challenges to survival, but underlying all of them is the constant threat of respiratory decompensation.

The problem divides readily into several individual entities for ease of discussion and understanding, but in the individual infant all aspects of the problem may be present concomitantly.

VENTILATION

Exchange of gases between the alveolar air sacs and the environment requires an unobstructed tubular passageway and the energy to perform the work required to achieve sufficient intrathoracic negative pressure to draw air into the lungs. Obstructions of the passageways may occur at several levels and may be congenital or acquired. Congenital anomalies causing airway obstruction include (a) choanal atresia, (b) pharyngeal malformations and tumors, (c) laryngeal abnormalities, and (d) tracheobronchial malformations. Acquired problems include (a) intubation injuries, (b) surgical procedures threatening airway patency or stability, (c) stenosis from prolonged intubations, (d) inflammatory diseases, (e) aspiration obstructions, and (f) tracheobronchial secretions obstructing the airway.

AIRWAY MANAGEMENT

This includes the use of tubes to maintain airway patency and stability and the use of mechanical ventilatory assistance to supply energy.

Indications for Intubation

These include the following: (a) mechanical obstructions to the airway, (b) inability to clear secretions, (c) the need for assisted ventilation by means of a respirator, and (d) the need for positive-pressure oxygen delivery not amenable to the use of nasal prongs.

Oral or nasal endotracheal intubation should be chosen first unless the larynx is obstructed. Once airway stability is achieved the indications for tracheostomy are the following:

1. Instability of the airway with transoral or transnasal intubation, that is, the baby who frequently is inadvertently extubated with resultant respiratory crises and arrests.
2. Inability to clear secretions adequately through transoral or transnasal endotracheal tubes.
3. The need for prolonged endotracheal intubation. This time limit is defined differently in each institution and is based on comparative experiences with tracheostomy complications, on the one hand, and subglottic stenoses from prolonged endotracheal intubation, on the other.
4. Persistent mechanical airway obstruction not readily correctable surgically and requiring discharge to home with an artificial airway.

Airway injuries from endotracheal intubation can be minimized by the following:[81]

1. The use of careful, gentle, knowledgeable intubation techniques
2. The use of tubes that are loosely fitting in the larynx
3. Either firm immobilization of the baby's head or elastic mobility of the tube connection to the ventilator, in either case avoiding pressure on the larynx from the tube
4. Continuous and sufficient delivery of mist to the tube and airway
5. The use of soft, plastic, noncuffed tubes inserted without a stylet
6. Appropriate changes of the tube
7. The use of gentle aseptic suctioning techniques

Proper Intubation Technique for an Infant

The infant should be positioned with his head slightly forward but his neck in neutral position (not excessively extended). This position has been described as that of "sniffing the morning air"[82] (Fig. 18).

The child should be well preoxygenated by mask breathing of 100 percent oxygen. Pharyngeal secretions should be aspirated.

A straight, short blade should be used on the laryngoscope. The infant's mouth is opened with the physician's left hand and the blade inserted, gently pushing the tongue to the left. When the uvula is seen, the tip of the blade is placed against it. If the laryngoscope handle is now pushed toward the far corner of the room (where ceiling and wall join), the epiglottis will come into view. Note that the laryngoscope is not "rocked" or levered into this position. It is achieved by pushing and lifting with the forearm with the wrist straight and stiff. Once the epiglottis is in view, it is simply lifted up with the tip of the blade, exposing the larynx. At this point moderate pressure on the cricoid region externally may aid exposure.

A straight, plastic, uncuffed endotracheal tube with an adaptor of the proper size is then inserted and held against the cords with gentle pressure

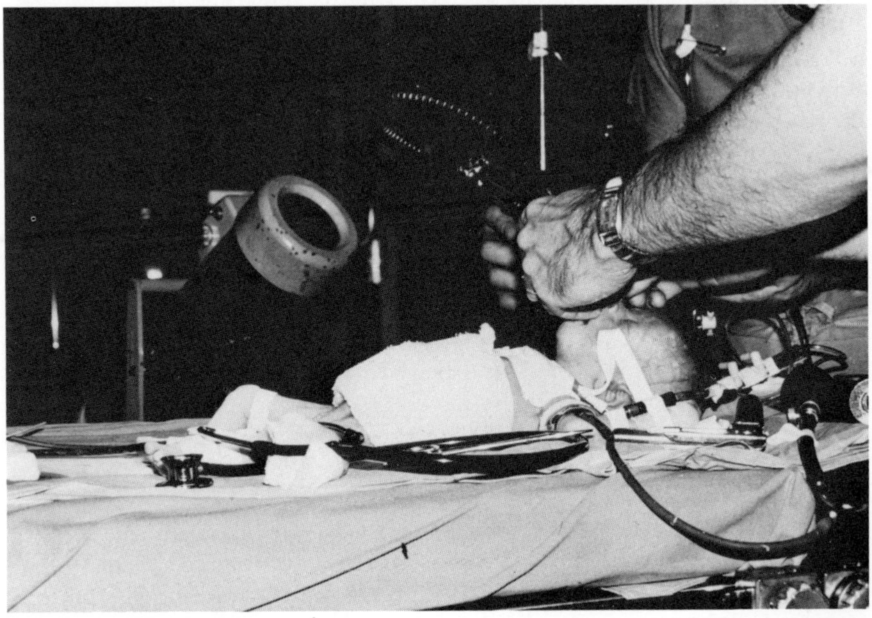

FIG.18. Infant in proper position for intubation. Note that head is slightly forward but not hyperextended.

until it passes into the trachea. Wetting the tube helps to ease its passage. Successful entry should be confirmed by direct visualization.

The above technique is that of Dr. Robert Crumrine, chief of pediatric anesthesia at Case Western Reserve University Hospitals. It has proved to be a most gentle one for the baby and an easy stepwise approach for teaching residents.

Tracheostomy

Tracheostomy has long been a highly valuable procedure for the management of airway problems in adults and older children, providing a means for safer respirator therapy and easy access to the airway for clearing secretions, as well as providing lifesaving bypassing of upper airway obstructions. Its use in infancy has been feared by many because of excessive complications and frequent prolonged inability to extubate the patient after the need for the tracheostomy has passed.[81]

The use of refined surgical techniques together with the newer plastic tubes and the superior evaluation of the tiny infant trachea provided by the superb optical system of the newborn bronchoscopes with the optical telescopes*[84] have now made both emergency and elective tracheostomy a safer and highly valuable procedure for even the tiniest premature infant (Fig. 19).

Recognition of the frequent presence of a stomal granuloma and its effects on the airway during deep inspiration has led to the development of a careful stepwise program for definitive treatment of the granuloma and formal surgical closure of the tracheal stoma. This program ensures that extubation can be achieved with a high success rate in even the tiniest infants.[83]

TECHNIQUE

1. If the baby is not already intubated, an oral endotracheal tube should be placed, and usually general anesthesia is used. The procedure is performed in the operating room.

2. A small roll should be placed beneath the child's shoulders, and the head should be allowed to fall back gently. Extreme extension should be avoided, however, as this will pull the thoracic trachea up into the neck and result in a stoma that is too low. Extubation may then occur when the head is flexed.

3. A small (1.5- to 2-cm) transverse incision is placed one finger breadth above the sternal notch. It is deepened transversely through the platysma, and then the remaining dissection is completed in the midline in a sagittal plane between the strap muscles and through the pretracheal fascia. Great care must be used, as each level is dissected to ensure that the trachea remains

*Karl Storz Endoscopy-America, Inc., Los Angeles, Calif.

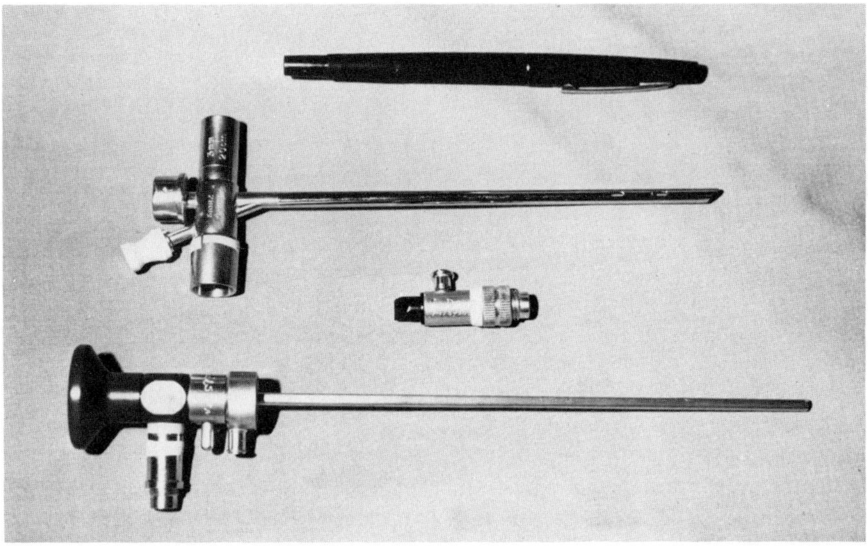

FIG.19. The optical telescopic bronchoscope for newborns. The sheath has an outer diameter of <3.5 mm. Superb optics, stable anesthetic control, and imaginative instrumentation possibilities combine to make this a very useful instrument for newborns.

in the midline and is not pulled to one side by the retractors. Palpation for the trachea above the incision helps to locate it. The isthmus of the thyroid should be identified and if necessary its inferior attachment to the trachea freed from the trachea and gently retracted cephalad.

4. Once the trachea is identified, it should be dissected sufficiently to allow placement of two silk sutures as far laterally as possible. These sutures will aid subsequently in replacing an inadvertently dislodged tube. By pulling them apart (toward the shoulders), the stoma will be opened and elevated toward the skin surface.

5. A midtracheal vertical slit incision is then made slightly longer than the diameter of the proposed tube. It should be tailored to admit the tube easily. If the tube has to be forced in or the stoma spread open with an instrument, tearing of the stoma may result in difficulties with subsequent closure and extubation.

6. A plastic tube (Silastic or polyvinyl chloride) of the Aberdeen design is then inserted.[85,86] The proper size will fill most of the tracheal lumen but will enter without friction or the need for undue force. Prior to insertion, of course, the oral endotracheal tube is withdrawn by the anesthesiologist until its tip can just be seen at the superior margin of the stoma.

7. Placement of the tube is facilitated by moistening it with sterile saline. It is inserted from the side, allowing its narrowed anteroposterior diameter at the tip to slide easily into the vertical slit stoma. The tube is then rotated 90 degrees to the proper alignment.

8. The tube is secured with cloth tape ties around the neck. An x-ray to ensure that the tip of the tube is above the carina is mandatory. The tube may have to be shortened in an occasional baby.

9. If the incision is of proper size, no closing sutures are required lateral to the tube. Bleeding in the midline dissection is minimal. With proper technique the overall dissection is so minimal that the incidence of postoperative subcutaneous or mediastinal emphysema is almost nonexistent.

SUBSEQUENT CARE

Continuous mist must be delivered to the plastic tubes, since they have no inner cannula to facilitate cleaning. If adequate mist and frequent, gentle suctioning are provided, the tubes remain very clean.[81] The tube is changed weekly and, at the first change, the lateral retention sutures are removed to avoid granuloma formation around them.

Wetting the new tubes prior to insertion is extremely important. If this is not done the tube may adhere to the stomal tract as it enters, rolling the skin in and obstructing the stoma in the trachea itself.

CLOSURE OF THE STOMA

When the need for the tracheostomy has passed, extubation can almost always be achieved if a carefully thought out program is adhered to. The following points are cogent:

1. The smallest tube available occupies so great a part of the infant's airway that the frequently used program of progressively smaller tubes and partial "corking" of the tube lumen, which is usually successful for older patients, is rarely successful in infancy.
2. If even a short period of oral or nasal endotracheal intubation occurred, laryngeal or subglottic stenosis may be present and must be ruled out before tracheal extubation is attempted.
3. The inspiratory collapse that occurs in the infant's trachea after removal of the tracheostomy tube is rarely due to "tracheomalacia," as has usually been alleged in the past, but to the presence of a lumen-narrowing granuloma on the inside of the trachea at the superior margin of the stoma.

The development of the newborn bronchoscope with optical telescope* provides the superb optical system that allows visualization of this tiny

*Karl Storz Endoscopy-America, Inc., Los Angeles, Calif.

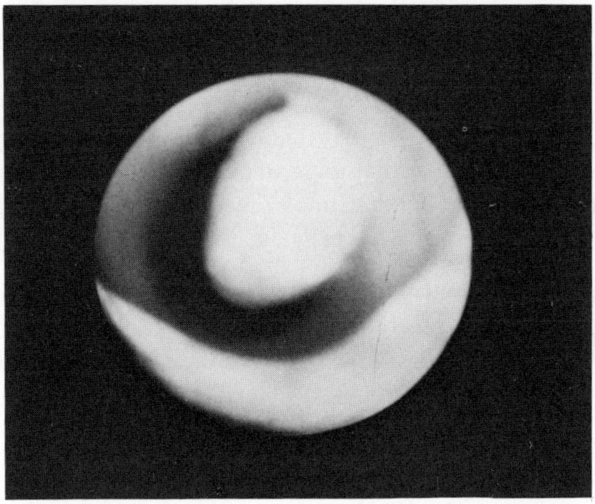

FIG.20. View of granuloma at the tracheal stoma site through the optical telescopic bronchoscope. (Courtesy of Dr. Dale G. Johnson).

granuloma as well as the opportunity to observe its effects on the airway lumen during inspiration (Fig.20).

The granuloma partially narrows the airway above the stoma so that, when the stoma collapses in after extubation and the child tries to inspire deeply, the airway obstructs at the granuloma and the stoma is sucked in, collapsing the trachea and further obstructing the tracheal lumen.

OUTLINE OF PROCEDURES FOR TRACHEAL EXTUBATION

1. Initial laryngoscopy and bronchoscopy with the newborn (3-mm) bronchoscope ensures that the airway is open, that no laryngeal or subglottic stenosis exists, that the cords function normally, and that the distal airway is clean, open, and free of secretions.
2. The tracheostomy tube is removed and the stoma carefully inspected with the bronchoscope for evidence of a granuloma at its inner superior margin. It is easily recognized if present.
3. If no granuloma is present, the tracheostomy tube is replaced, the child allowed to awaken thoroughly from anesthesia, and the tube then removed in the recovery room or intensive care area with provisions for adequate prolonged observation. Usually rapid functional stomal closure and continued lumen patency are achieved.
4. If a granuloma is present, preparation is made for operative closure of the stoma. The child is intubated with an oral endotracheal tube. The tracheostomy tube is removed, and the neck is prepped and draped.

a. An elliptical transverse incision is made in the skin around the stoma and deepened through to the trachea, essentially "coring" out the stoma.

b. When the trachea is identified, the dissection is continued toward the stoma until the actual edge of the incision in the trachea itself is identified and freed of stomal scar tissue all the way around its perimeter.

c. The external stomal tract now exists as a tube-like projection surrounded by the edge of the original tracheal incision and in continuity with the granuloma on the inner superior margin of the stoma in the trachea itself.

d. Using a small, narrow dental dissector or similar instrument, careful separation of the stomal tract from the edge of the tracheal incision is achieved. This dissection is continued on the under side of the superior margin of the stoma separating the granuloma from the tracheal inner wall.

e. The granuloma then can be easily lifted out with the attached contiguous stomal tract (Fig.21), leaving a clean tracheal incision and lumen. Gentle probing of the tracheal inner wall above the stoma with a small curved mosquito hemostat insures that all the granuloma has been removed.

f. Since the original incision in the tracheal wall was a simple vertical slit, what remains is a clean-edged, narrow, vertical elliptical tracheal stoma. This is then easily sutured closed with four or five

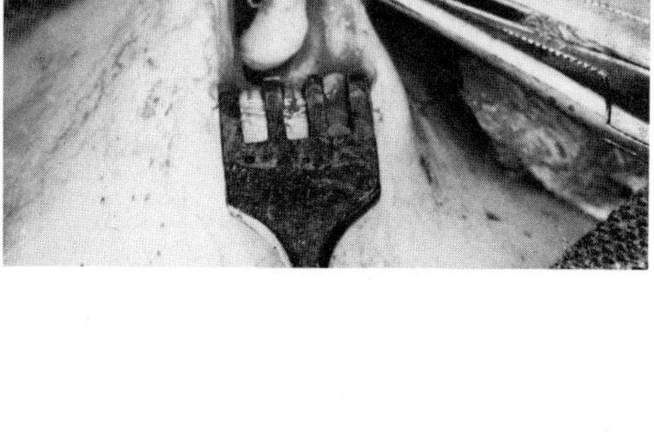

FIG.21. The granuloma at the tracheal stoma site being removed with the stomal tract. (Photograph courtesy of Dr. Dale Johnson).

simple sutures of 4/0 chromic catgut, restoring the structural strength of the tracheal "arch" at the stoma site and helping to prevent collapse inward with deep inspiration.

g. Layered closure of the strap muscles and fascial tissues in the midline with chromic catgut further supports the airway. The skin is usually left open and packed with a small wick soaked in antiseptic solution* to obviate subcutaneous infection. It closes readily after the packing is removed a few days later.

5. The child is then allowed to awaken thoroughly from anesthesia before extubation. If he is too agitated he is given morphine sulfate, 0.05 mg/kg, after insuring that his agitation is not due to hypoxia.
6. After prolonged skilled nursing and medical observation has been provided for, the endotracheal tube is removed and the child carefully observed.
7. Adequate mist therapy must be continued, usually in the form of ultrasonic nebulization to provide continued liquidity of tracheobronchial secretions.

Dr. Dale Johnson has perfected a method for endoscopic resection of the granuloma utilizing the infant optical resectoscope. This procedure obviates the need for formal surgical excision of the granuloma.[82]

FOLLOW-UP CARE

The child is gradually weaned from mist therapy over the next several days. Occasionally reintubation and suctioning with an oral endotracheal tube may be required if secretions prove to be more tenacious or abundant than anticipated. The tube is removed immediately after each suctioning episode (after adequate ventilation with oxygen, of course).

When the child is well stabilized and ready for discharge, bronchoscopy is again performed to insure that no new granuloma is forming at the stomal closure site. This is usually done one week following extubation. Once recovered from this procedure, the child can be safely discharged.

MECHANICAL VENTILATION

Introduction

Mechanical ventilation is required when the infant can no longer successfully ventilate himself. The primary indication for use of a ventilator is a ris-

*Betadine Solution, Purdue Frederick Co., Norwalk, Conn.

ing PCO_2 and falling pH in a baby with a clear airway. Causes of ventilatory insufficiency are the following:

1. Cerebral—depression of respiratory center by
   a. Apnea of newborn
   b. Sepsis
   c. Intracranial hemorrhage
   d. Severe acidosis
   e. Intracranial mass lesions
2. Respiratory—mechanical
   a. Stiff lungs (edema, pneumonia)
   b. Pneumothorax
   c. Chest wall compression
   d. Decreased diaphragmatic excursion due to
      (1) Abnormalities of diaphragm
      (2) Increased intra-abdominal pressure
      (3) Extrinsic abdominal compression
3. Systemic—inability of infant to perform normal work of breathing
   a. Debility, nutritional deficiency
   b. Extreme prematurity
   c. Severe generalized sepsis
   d. Metabolic derangements

When PCO_2 approaches a level of 55 mm Hg, ventilatory assistance should be initiated. Leaving a tiring baby struggling without help is inviting insidious hypoxia, respiratory arrest, and catastrophe.

Ventilators

Various ventilators are adaptable to infants but should have at least the following characteristics:

1. Ability to deliver small, dependable volumes of gases. An infant requires 7 to 10 ml of gas per kilogram for tidal volume from the ventilator. Normal tidal volume of a newborn is about 6 ml of gas per kilogram.[87]

2. Volume-controlled delivery. The respirator must be able to increase pressure to deliver the desired volume.

3. Pressure warning system. It should be possible to set the machine to warn if it must raise pressure above a safe preset point to deliver the required volume. Usually 40 to 45 mm Hg is the chosen pressure limit.

4. Easy gas mixture to achieve desired O_2 concentrations.

5. Adaptability to positive airway pressure methods.

6. Ability to provide both controlled, assisted, and intermittent or partially controlled ventilation. This greatly facilitates weaning the child from the ventilator.

OXYGENATION

INTRODUCTION

The delivery of oxygen to the pulmonary capillaries obviously requires that it be delivered to the alveoli. In this sense it is not independent of ventilation. However, once adequate ventilation is achieved, oxygenation becomes an entity independent of the ventilatory problem. Adequate oxygenation requires that oxygen in the alveolus be able to diffuse to the capillaries in sufficient concentration to maintain a gradient from the blood to the tissues so that oxygen will diffuse from the blood to the tissues.

Any factor preventing any given volume of pulmonary capillary blood from acquiring its content of oxygen will contribute to dilution of systemic arterial blood by unoxygenated blood. This can occur under the following conditions:

1. A section of lung that is perfused by blood is not being ventilated at the alveolar level.

2. Oxygen cannot diffuse from the alveolus to the capillary because of edema or inflammation in the interstitium.

3. Pulmonary arterial blood is shunted to the venous outflow at the precapillary level.

4. The binding of oxygen to hemoglobin is blocked, as in carbon monoxide poisoning.

CORRECTION OF DEFICIENCIES

Oxygenation deficiencies can usually be corrected by[87–90](a) increasing the percentage of oxygen in the inspired gases or (b) increasing the pressure at which oxygen is delivered to the alveolar capillary interface. This is usually achieved by increasing the mean pressure of the respiratory cycle using either continuous positive airway pressure[89] or positive end expiratory pressure. Both approaches essentially work by eliminating the usual low pressure gradient of the expiratory phase. Usually CPAP is delivered by tube without a ventilator, whereas PEEP is used in conjunction with mechanical ventilation.

The choice between increasing oxygen percentage and increasing mean cycle pressure is based on an estimate of where the problem lies. Insufficient alveolar ventilation can often be overcome with positive pressure alone; transmembrane diffusion difficulties secondary to edema can occasionally be overcome in the same manner. It has been suggested that all infants that are intubated should be maintained on 2 to 3 cm H_2O positive pressure because bypassing the glottic valsalva mechanism with the tube may lead to atelectasis and alveolar hypoventilation.[91] Higher levels of either inspired oxygen concentration or positive pressure may lead to deleterious side effects.[75,92]

As pressure is increased, the gradient between alveolar partial pressures and capillary partial pressures is increased, facilitating gas diffusion. However, the negative pressure of inspiration is lessened, decreasing venous return to the heart and reducing cardiac output. In a baby with normal lung compliance, increased ventilatory pressure may therefore reduce oxygenation at the tissue level due to reduced blood flow and perfusion pressure.

On the other hand, high levels of inspired oxygen are directly toxic to the alveolar membranes, leading eventually to alveolar fibrosis and bronchopulmonary dysplasia.[75,92] This converts acute pulmonary insufficiency to a chronic debility state. Pulmonary vascular hypertension may result, and eventual right heart failure (cor pulmonale) may occur.

Infants with marked reductions of lung compliance may tolerate high pressures very well. Generally, when high levels of both inspired oxygen and pressure are used concomitantly, it is best to reduce inspired oxygen below 80 percent first, then try to reduce positive pressure below 10 cm H_2O, and then further reduce inspired O_2 below 40 percent. Pressure can then be reduced to 5 cm H_2O and then O_2 tapered back to room air before discontinuing the pressure altogether. Hall and Rhodes have reported pneumothorax and pneumomediastinum in *improving* infants who previously tolerated high airway pressures. As lung compliance improves, rupture occurs. Therefore, pressure must be reduced along with O_2 concentration.[93] Incremental reductions of O_2 should not exceed 5 percent and pressure reduction increments should be no more than 2 cm H_2O.

Obviously, each step must be diligently monitored by means of arterial blood gases. Remember that either increased pressure or increased inspired O_2 concentrations can lead to PO_2 levels in excess of 100 mm Hg and produce retrolental fibroplasia.

PHARMACOLOGIC MANIPULATIONS

Fluid Restriction and Albumin Therapy

When edema due to decreased intravascular oncotic pressure is the cause of oxygenation difficulties, restriction of intravenously administered fluids combined with bolus injections of 25 percent salt-poor albumin, 4 ml/kg every 6 to 8 hours, will reverse the gradient and cause fluid to move from the pulmonary interstitium to the vascular space.

Diuretics

If the above regimen fails to increase urinary excretion or if fluid in the pulmonary interstitium is not the result of intravascular albumin deficiency, furosemide can be used to force a diuresis. This will lower intravascular hydrostatic pressure and allow fluid resorption from the pulmonary interstitium. Refer to the section in Chapter 3, Section I, on central venous pressure monitoring before undertaking this step.

Myocardial Stimulants

When myocardial insufficiency may be playing the primary role in interstitial edema, digitalization will improve cardiac output, decrease venous pressure, and reverse the hydrostatic gradient to favor fluid resorption. As noted elsewhere, dopamine is probably a better choice, since it stimulates myocardial contractility and improves cardiac output without the risk of arrhythmias attendant on the use of digitalis. In addition, improved renal perfusion is directly achieved and diuresis will usually occur.

Recent interest in the use of pulmonary vasodilators such as tolazoline* and chlorpromazine† may prove to be useful in severe pulmonary hypertensive states such as bronchopulmonary dysplasias and postoperative diaphragmatic hernias.[59]

*Priscoline, CIBA Pharmaceutical Co., Summit, N.J.
†Thorazine, Smith, Kline, and French Laboratories, Philadelphia, Pa.

APPENDIX

DIGITALIZATION SCHEDULE

1. Drug of choice: Digoxin
2. Dosage:
   a. Initial digitalization for newborn infants
      (1) Slowly—0.06 mg/kg total in three doses. Usually one-half the dose, then one-fourth the dose every 6 hours × 2 doses. The schedule is the same for intramuscular or intravenous administration.
      (2) More rapidly—0.04 mg/kg total in three doses. One-half the total dose, then one-fourth the dose every 3 hours × 2 doses.
      (3) In early infancy the dose then rises to 0.08 mg/kg total for digitalizing.
      (4) Later in childhood the dose gradually falls back to 0.02 to 0.03 mg/kg total for digitalization.
   b. Maintenance: One-eighth of the digitalizing dose every 12 hours.

GUIDELINE FOR ANTIBIOTIC DOSAGE

1. Parenteral
   a. Penicillin: 50 to 100,000 units/kg per day in four doses
   b. Ampicillin: 100 to 400 mg/kg per day in four doses (average 200 mg/kg per day)

c. Keflin: 150 to 180 mg/kg per day in four doses

d. Polymyxin B: 5 to 8 mg/kg per day IV or IM in three doses

e. Gentamycin: 3 to 8 mg/kg per day IV in three divided doses or IM for neonates; 3 to 5 mg/kg per day for infants and older; maintain good urine output; monitor serum levels

f. Kanamycin: 15 mg/kg per day IM in two doses

2. Oral

a. Penicillin or ampicillin: 125 mg q.i.d.

b. Gantrisin: 100 mg/kg per day in four doses (may be given IM)

c. Lipogantrisin: 100 to 200 mg/kg per day in two doses

3. Antibiotic dosage for gastrointestinal preparation preoperatively

a. Kanamycin (oral): 15 mg/kg per day in four doses for one to three days

b. Neomycin: 50 mg/kg per day in four to six doses for one to three days

c. Nonabsorbable sulfas: 100 to 200 mg/kg per day in same divisions as neomycin
Note: The *Physicians Desk Reference* in general gives inadequate dosage levels for children's antibiotics. For doses of drugs other than the above consult a handbook of pediatrics.

GUIDELINE FOR ORAL ALIMENTATION REQUIREMENTS

1. Newborns and infants

a. Water: 150 ml/kg per day

b. Calories: 100 cal/kg per day

c. Upper limit is 32 oz of formula (960 ml); initially six feedings; drop to five by 1 month and four by 2 months

2. Basic infant formulas in use

   a. Enfamil*or Similac† (a standard nutrient milk formula attempting to approximate human breast milk)

      (1) E20—20 cal/oz
      (2) E13—13 cal/oz
      (3) E24—24 cal/oz
      (4) E24—with iron

   b. Nutramigen*: 20 cal/oz (casein hydrolysate); consists of protein hydrolysates requiring less digestion and leaving less residue; better tolerated for early feedings after gastrointestinal surgery and useful as regular feedings for cystic fibrosis babies; contains sucrose and is lactose free.

   c. Probana*: 20 cal/oz; made from banana powder, a time-honored remedy for infant diarrheas; useful for patients with short bowel syndrome or postsurgical frequency of stool; particularly useful for intractable diarrhea after resection surgery, especially for NEC; this is not a simple formula, however

   d. Pregestimil*: 20 cal/oz; the most basic formula made up of glucose and protein hydrolysates and medium-chain triglycerides requiring very little digestion

3. Other oral requirements

   a. Vitamins

      (1) Tri-Vi-Sol 1.0 ml maintenance
      (2) Poly-Vi-Sol 1.0 ml after 6 months

   b. Iron
      (1) Fer-In-Sol 1.0 ml gives 25 mg elemental iron

   c. Solids: Usually begun at about 4 weeks of age, but sooner if weight gain inadequate on full formula; start with rice cereal for its low allergenic properties and add one food at a time

4. Advancing feedings: The simplest way to accomplish this is to always offer the infant a little more in the bottle than he took the previous feeding. In this way the baby will gradually consume more per feeding and eventually increase the interval between feedings until a feeding is "dropped".

*Mead Johnson Laboratories, Evansville, Ind.
†Ross Laboratories, Columbus, Ohio

OUTLINE OF INSTRUCTIONS TO BE GIVEN REFERRING PHYSICIANS AND INFORMATION TO BE OBTAINED FROM THEM

1. Information to be obtained

   a. Patient's name, age, location.

   b. Physician's name, address, and telephone (office and home).

   c. Hospital location and phone.

   d. Suspected diagnosis.

   e. Medications given to date (especially type of vitamin K).

   f. Results: x-ray, lab work, etc.

   g. Observations of baby's stool, urine, vomitus (note quantity, character, and color).

   h. Applicable family history.

   i. Plans for transport and estimate of when baby will be ready to travel.

   j. Maternal history: hydramnios, toxemia, infection, miscarriages, medication, and weight gain.

2. Advice to be given to referring physicians

   a. They are responsible until baby is safely transported. Decision to transport and responsibility for it is theirs.

   b. Must keep neonates warm—incubator, warm car, aluminum foil wrap, etc.

   c. Give 1 mg Aquamephyton.

   d. Send sample 10 ml of mother's blood (in case of need for exchange transfusion) in plain tube.

   e. Should not routinely start IV.

   f. Baby should have nasogastric tube in place with two extra holes and with constant suction during the trip. An 8 French rubber catheter with extra holes in the distal 3 cm works well.

   g. Start antibiotics if the situation requires (gastroschises).

   h. Send signed operative permit (cross out referring hospital name and substitute medical center) unless parent accompanying.

i. Send the father.

j. Send x-rays, lab results, chart information (ensure that x-rays will be returned).

k. Thank the referring physician and assure him that continued information and reports will be sent to him.

3. Special cases

a. Diaphragmatic hernia: Get blood gases as emergency; do not intubate if can be avoided; warn about pneumothorax if tubed; keep warm. Put nasogastric tube down and ensure its continued function.

b. Tracheoesophageal fistula: Good suction in proximal pouch; prone position, head elevated 45 degrees; no radiographic contrast.

c. Omphaloceles, gastroschises, sacrococcygeal teratomas: Cover with sterile saline-soaked gauze; start antibiotics in recommended doses; nasogastric tubes. Check with surgical visitant prior to transfer for further suggestions.

REFERENCES

1. Moore FD: Metabolic Care of the Surgical Patient. Philadelphia, Saunders, 1959, p 292
2. Wright HK, Gann DS, Drucker WR: Current concepts of therapy for derangements of extracellular fluid. In Davis JH (ed): Current Concepts in Surgery. New York, McGraw-Hill, 1965
3. Shires T, Williams J, Brown F: Acute change in ECF associated with major surgical procedures. Ann Surg 154:803, 1961
4. Weil MH, Shubin H: Diagnosis and Treatment of Shock. Baltimore, Williams & Wilkins, 1967, p 122
5. Strauss MB: Body Water in Man. Boston, Little, Brown, 1957. Referenced in Davis JH (ed): Current Concepts in Surgery. New York, McGraw-Hill, 1965
6. Wright HK, Gann DS: Correction of defect in free water excretion in postoperative patients by extracellular fluid volume expansion. Ann Surg 158:70, 1963
7. Share L: Acute reduction in extracellular fluid volume and concentration of antidiuretic hormone in blood. Endocrinology 69:925, 1961
8. Wright HK, Gann DS: On the mechanism by which acute ECF expansion promotes Na excretion. Clin Res 11:254, 1963
9. Moore FD, Shires GT: Moderation. Ann Surg 166:300, 1967
10. Rickham PP: Preoperative and postoperative care: neonates. In Mustard WT, Ravitch MM, Snyder WH, Jr., et al (eds): Pediatric Surgery. Chicago, Year Book, 1969, p 38
11. Rickham PP: The metabolic response to neonatal surgery. Cambridge, Harvard Univ Press, 1957
12. Wilkinson AW, Nagy G, Billing BH, et al: Excretion of chloride and sodium after operation. Lancet I:640, 1949
13. Kaplan SA: Fluid and electrolyte therapy: maintenance, abnormal states, methods of administration. Pediatr Clin North Am 16:581, 1969
14. Dibbins AW, Kiesewetter WB: Preoperative and postoperative care: infants and children. In Mustard WT, Ravitch MM, Snyder WH, Jr., et al (eds):Pediatric Surgery, Chicago, Year Book, 1969, p 54
15. Rowe MI, Arango A: The neonatal response to massive fluid infusion. J. Pediatr Surg 6:365, 1971
16. Colle E, Paulsen E: Response of the newborn infant to major surgery: effects on water, electrolyte, and nitrogen balance. Pediatrics 23:1063, 1959
17. Wallace WM: Quantitative requirements of the infant and child for water and electrolyte under varying conditions. Am J Clin Pathol 23:1133, 1953
18. Crumrine RS: Postoperative hypoxia in infants and children. Int Anesthesiol Clin 9:83, 1971
19. Verney EB: Antidiuretic hormone and the factors which determine its release. Proc R Soc Lond SB 135:25, 1947–1948. Cited in Wright HK, Gann DS, Drucker WR: Current concepts of therapy for derangements of extracellular fluid. In Davis JH (ed): Current Concepts in Surgery. New York, McGraw-Hill, 1965
20. Weil MH, Shubin H: Diagnosis and Treatment of Shock. Baltimore, Williams & Wilkins, 1967, p 88

21. Drucker WR, Wright HK: Physiology and pathophysiology of gastrointestinal fluids. In Ravitch MM (ed): Current Problems in Surgery. Chicago, Year Book, 1964, p 23
22. Hoye RC, Bennett SH, Geelhoed GW, et al: Fluid volume and albumin knetics occurring with major surgery. JAMA 222:1255, 1972
23. Giordano JM, Joseph WL, Klingenmeier CH, et al: The management of interstitial pulmonary edema, significance of hypoproteinemia. J Thorac Cardiovasc Surg 64:739, 1972
24. Moylan FMB, O'Connell KC, Todres ID, et al: Edema of the pulmonary interstitium in infants and children. Pediatrics 55:783, 1975
25. Moss GS, Siegel DC, Cochin MS, et al: Effects of saline and colloid solutions on pulmonary function in hemorrhagic shock. Surg Gynecol Obstet 133:53, 1971
26. Tullis JL: Albumin 1. Background and use. JAMA 237:355, 1977
27. Holcroft JW, Trunkey DD: Pulmonary extravasation of albumin during and after hemorrhagic shock in baboons. J Surg Res 18:91, 1975
28. Tullis JL: Albumin 2. Guidelines for clinical use. JAMA 237:460, 1977
29. Kukral JC, Brandly JM, Fritsch BA, et al: Total body composition in cirrhotic patients with metabolic alkalosis, hypokalemia, hyperammonemia and portacaval shunt. Am J Surg 117: 85, 1969
30. Gross S, Melhorn D: Exchange transfusion with citrated whole blood for disseminated intravascular coagulation. J Pediatr 78:415, 1971
31. Hutter JJ, Hathaway WE, Wayne ER: Hematologic abnormalities in neonatal necrotizing enterocolitis. J Pediatr 88:1026, 1976
32. Holden WD, Krieger H, Levey S, et al: The effect of nutrition on nitrogen metabolism in the surgical patient. Ann Surg 146:563, 1957
33. Riegel C, Rhoads JE, Koop CE, et al: Dietary requirements for nitrogen equilibrium in the period immediately following certain major surgical operations. Am J Med Sci 210:133, 1945.
34. Dudrick SJ, Rhoads JE, Vars HM: Growth of puppies receiving all nutritional requirements by vein. Fortschr Parenter Ernahrung 2:16, 1967
35. Dudrick SJ, Wilmore DW, Vars HM, et al: Long-term total parenteral nutrition with growth, development and positive nitrogen balance. Surgery 64:134, 1968
36. Wilmore DW, Dudrick SJ: Growth and development of an infant receiving all nutrients exclusively by vein. JAMA 203:860, 1968
37. Dudrick SJ, Wilmore DW, Vars HM: Can intravenous feeding as the sole means of nutrition support growth in the child and restore weight loss in an adult? Ann Surg 169:974, 1969
38. Wilmore DW, Groff DB, Bishop HC, et al: Total parenteral nutrition in infants with catastrophic gastrointestinal anomalies. J Pediatr Surg 4:181, 1969
39. Wilmore DW: Factors correlating with a successful outcome following extensive intestinal resection in newborn infants. J Pediatr 80:88, 1972
40. Filler RM, Eraklis AJ, Rubin VG, et al: Long-term total parenteral nutrition in infants. N Engl J Med 281:589, 1969
41. Groff DB, Ahmed N: Subclavian vein catheterization in the infant. J Pediatr Surg 9:171, 1974
42. Morgan WW, Jr., Harkins GA: Percutaneous introduction of long-term indwelling venous catheters in infants. J Pediatr Surg 7:538, 1972

43. Boeckman CR, Krill CE: Bacterial and fungal infections complicating parenteral alimentation in infants and children. J Pediatr Surg 5:117, 1970
44. Stone HH: Studies in the pathogenesis, diagnosis and treatment of candida sepsis in children. J Pediatr Surg 9:127, 1974
45. Miller RC, Grogan JB: Incidence and source of contamination of intravenous nutritional infusion systems. J Pediatr Surg 8:185, 1973
46. Groff DB: Complications of intravenous hyperalimentation in newborns and infants. J Pediatr Surg 4:460, 1969
47. Bryan H, Shennan A, Griffin A, et al: Intralipid—Its rational use in parenteral nutrition of the newborn. Pediatrics 58:787, 1976
48. Heird WC, Winters RW: Total parenteral nutrition, the state of the art. J Pediatr 86:2, 1975
49. Driscoll JM, Jr, Heird WC, Schullinger JN, et al: Total intravenous alimentation in low-birthweight infants— a preliminary report. J Pediatr 81:145, 1972
50. Coran AG: Total intravenous feeding of infants and children without the use of a central venous catheter. Ann Surg 179:445, 1974
51. Touloukian RJ, Seashore JH: Hepatic secretory obstruction with total parenteral nutrition in the infant. J Pediatr Surg 10:353, 1975
52. Gutenberger JE, Miller DL, Dibbons AW, et al: Hypogammaglobulinemia and hypoalbuminemia in neonates with ruptured omphaloceles and gastroschisis. J Pediatr Surg 8:353, 1973
53. Klaus MH, Fanaroff AA: Care of the High-Risk Neonate. Philadelphia, Saunders, 1973
54. Klaus MH, Fanaroff AA: The physical environment. In Klaus MH, Fanaroff AA (eds): Care of the High-Risk Neonate. Philadelphia, Saunders, 1973, pp 59, 60, 68
55. Downes JJ: Resuscitation and intensive care of the newborn. Int Anesthesiol Clin 6:911, 1968
56. Adams F, Lind J: Physiologic studies on the cardiovascular status of normal newborn infants, with special reference to the ductus arteriosus. Pediatrics 19:431, 1957
57. Edmunds LH, Jr, Downes JJ: Assisted ventilation of infants. In Sabiston DC, Jr, Spencer FC (eds): Gibbon's Surgery of the Chest. Philadelphia, Saunders, 1976, p 226
58. Liebman J, Whitman V: The heart. In Klaus MH, Fanaroff AA (eds): Care of the High-Risk Neonate. Philadelphia, Saunders, 1973, p 236
59. Dibbons AW, Weiner ES: Mortality from neonatal diaphragmatic hernia. J Pediatr Surg 9:653, 1974
60. Fisher D, Behrman RE: Resuscitation of the newborn infant. In Klaus MH, Fanaroff AA (eds): Care of the High-Risk Neonate. Philadelphia, Saunders, 1973, p 3
61. Srouji MN: The acid-base status of the surgical neonate on admission to the hospital. Surgery 62:958, 1967
62. Beckwith JB: Extreme cytomegaly of the adrenal fetal cortex, omphalocele, hyperplasia of kidneys and pancreas, and Leydig-cell hyperplasia—another syndrome? Presented at the Annual Meeting of Western Society for Pediatric Research, Los Angeles, Nov 11, 1963
63. Benson CD, Lloyd JR: The small intestine. Atresia and stenosis of the jejunum and ileum. In Mustard WT, Ravitch MM, Snyder WH, Jr, et al (eds): Pediatric Surgery. Chicago, Year Book, 1969, p 845
64. Woolley MM, Felsher BF, Asch MJ, et al: Jaundice, hypertrophic pyloric stenosis, and hepatic glucuronyl transferase. J Pediatr Surg 9:359, 1974

65. Chaves-Carballo E, Harris LE, Lynn HB: Jaundice associated with pyloric stenosis and neonatal small-bowel obstructions. Clin Pediatr 7:198, 1968
66. Filston HC, Johnson DG: Percutaneous venous cannulation in neonates and infants: a method for catheter insertion without "cut-down." Pediatrics 48:896, 1971
67. Vidyasagar D, Downes JJ, Boggs TR: Respiratory distress syndrome of newborn infants, II. Technic of catheterization of umbilical artery and clinical results of treatment of 124 patients. Clin Pediatr 9:332, 1970
68. Filston HC, Izant RJ, Jr: Translocation of the umbilical artery to the lower abdomen: an adjunct to the postoperative monitoring of arterial blood gases in major abdominal wall defects. J Pediatr Surg 10:225, 1975
69. Johnson DG, Ito T: Continuous flush of arterial pressure recording catheters. J Thorac Cardiovasc Surg 57:675, 1969
70. Noblett HR: Treatment of uncomplicated meconium ileus by Gastrografin enema: a preliminary report. J Pediatr Surg 4:190, 1969
71. Wagget J, Johnson DG, Borns P, et al: The non-operative treatment of meconium ileus by Gastrografin enema. J Pediatr 77:407, 1970
72. Rowe MI, Seagram G, Weinberger M: Gastrografin induced hypertonicity: the pathogenesis of a neonatal hazard. Am J Surg 125:185, 1973
73. Fanaroff AA, Klaus M: Neonatal infections. In Klaus M, Fanaroff AA (eds): Care of the High-Risk Neonate. Philadelphia, Saunders, 1973
74. Raflo GT, Jones RCW, Jr, Wangensteen SL: Inadequacy of steroids in treatment of severe hemorrhagic shock. Am J Surg 130:321, 1975
75. Klaus M, Fanaroff AA: Respiratory problems. In Klaus M, Fanaroff AA (eds): Care of the High-Risk Neonate. Philadelphia, Saunders, 1973
76. Goetzman BW, Stadalnik RC, Bogren HG, et al: Thrombotic complications of umbilical artery catheters. Pediatrics 56:374, 1975
77. Gauderer M, Holgersen LO: Peripheral arterial line insertion in neonates and infants: a simplified method of temporal artery cannulation. J Pediatr Surg 9:875, 1974
78. Prian GW: New proximal approach works well in temporal artery catheterization. JAMA 235:2693, 1976
79. Weil MH, Shubin H: Diagnosis and treatment of shock. Baltimore, Williams & Wilkins, 1967, p 273
80. Talbert JL, Haller JA: The optimal site for central venous measurement in newborn infants. J Surg Res 6:168, 1966
81. Lindholm C: Prolonged endotracheal intubation. Acta Anaesthesiol Scand [Suppl] 33:1, 1969
82. Johnson DG, Jones R: Surgical aspects of airway management in infants and children. Surg Clin North Am 56:263, 1976
83. Filston HC, Johnson DG, Crumrine RS: Infant tracheostomy: a new look with a solution to the difficult decannulation problem. Am J Dis Child (submitted for publication).
84. Gans SL, Berci G: Advances in endoscopy in infants and children. J Pediatr Surg 6:199, 1971
85. Aberdeen EL: Tracheostomy and tracheostomy care in infants. Proc R Soc Med 58:900, 1965
86. Stool SE, Campbell JR, Johnson DG: Tracheostomy in children—the use of plastic tubes. J Pediatr Surg 3:402, 1968

87. Edmunds LH, Jr, Downes JJ: Assisted ventilation in infants. In Sabiston DC, Jr, Spencer FC (eds): Gibbon's Surgery of the Chest. Philadelphia, Saunders, 1976, p 227

88. Llewellyn A, Swyer P: Assisted ventilation. In Klaus MH, Fanaroff AA (eds): Care of the High-Risk Neonate. Philadelphia, Saunders, 1973

89. Gregory G, Kitterman J, Phibbs R, et al: Treatment of the idiopathic respiratory distress syndrome with continuous positive airway pressure. N Engl J Med 284:1333, 1971

90. Haller JA, Jr, White JJ, Moynihan PC, et al: Use of continuous positive airway pressure breathing in the improved management of neonatal emergencies. J Pediatr Surg 8:669, 1973

91. Fox WW, Berman LS, Dinwiddie R: Tracheal extubation of the neonate at 2 to 3 cm. H_2O continuous positive airway pressure. Pediatrics 59:257, 1977

92. Rhodes PG, Hall RT, Leonidas JC: Chronic pulmonary disease in neonates with assisted ventilation. Pediatrics 55:788, 1975

93. Hall RT, Rhodes PG: Pneumothorax and pneumomediastinum in infants with idiopathic respiratory distress syndrome receiving continuous positive airway pressure. Pediatrics 55:493, 1975

SECTION 2

RECOGNITION OF MAJOR NEWBORN CONGENITAL ANOMALIES

Without any question, the major factor in diagnosing a congenital anomaly is to keep the possibility of one occurring foremost in mind. The greatest delay in diagnosis is the result either of physicians attributing early signs and symptoms to normal variations or of ignoring them completely. If every child who presents with signs or symptoms that might be related to a congenital anomaly were immediately evaluated thoroughly enough to rule out the presence of an anomaly, many more of these children could be saved and many of those saved would have less complicated courses.

Next in importance is to know how anomalies present. What are the signs and symptoms? The earliest sign of many serious anomalies is hydramnios in the mother.[1,2] An infant whose mother had hydramnios should be immediately suspect and examined quickly and thoroughly, and baseline x-rays with appropriate follow-up should be obtained. Hydramnios represents a failure of the amniotic fluid to complete its normal pathway through the infant. The fluid ordinarily passes along the intestine of the infant, is resorbed to the infant's circulation, and is excreted by the infant kidney back into the amniotic fluid pool. An intestinal blockage above the midjejunum prevents resorption and leads to a backing up of fluid, which increases the amniotic fluid pool.

Finally, knowledge of the chronology of normal postnatal events is helpful. For example, with a normal neonate's first cry, air fills the stomach. With the next breath air enters the duodenum. By the end of 6 hours of extrauterine life, air should have reached the cecum. It may take up to 24 hours for air to reach the rectum, however. From this it is obvious that in a suspect neonate plain recumbent and erect films of the abdomen at 1 and 6 hours of life will usually show cardinal signs of abnormality, often before either vomiting or significant abdominal distention occurs. Thus, there is little excuse for not confirming the diagnosis of most neonatal intestinal obstructions in the first 12 hours of life. The failure to pass urine or meconium by 24 hours should in itself raise suspicion of anomaly and initiate investigation.[3]

Sepsis, disseminated intravascular coagulopathy, hypothermia, aspiration pneumonia, and distended and ischemic bowel are often more the result of iatrogenic delay than of a morphogenic error.

The initial discussions of this section outline the major congenital anomalies categorized by their presenting symptom complexes. The major anomalies in each group, especially those that are most lethal, are discussed in detail with emphasis on differential diagnosis and the most logical and safest courses of therapy. Nonsurgical disease presents identical or similar symptom complexes, and it is the rapid differentiation of the surgically amenable lesions from the nonsurgical that can salvage a good baby when even minimal delay in diagnosis and treatment may result in permanent debility, prolonged morbidity, and frequently death.

Most major newborn congenital anomalies can be placed into one of five presenting complexes: (a) signs of respiratory distress, (b) signs of gastrointestinal obstruction, (c) abdominal masses, (d) grossly obvious anomalies, and (e) bleeding. Each of these is presented in detail.

CHAPTER 1

CONGENITAL ANOMALIES THAT PRESENT WITH RESPIRATORY DISTRESS

INTRODUCTION

The key to successful diagnosis of any neonatal respiratory distress problem is a proper chest x-ray done the instant the subtlest of signs or symptoms is noted. No newborn nursery is properly equipped unless at least a portable x-ray machine and a knowledgeable operator are immediately available. Too often oxygen administration is used in lieu of rapid diagnostic evaluation because of convenience and because the symptom complex is assumed to be hyaline membrane disease. Remember that oxygen is to respiratory distress as aspirin is to a headache. Each treats a symptom without seeking an etiology.

Of the common symptoms of respiratory distress, restlessness is the least emphasized, the most difficult to detect, and the hardest to demonstrate to others. However, it is the first significant sign. A neonate in progressive respiratory distress starts first by being restless, then tachypneic; retraction follows and finally cyanosis. Naturally, in acute respiratory distress, all signs may begin simultaneously. Signs and symptoms alone, however, give no clue to etiology.

The chest x-ray, in most instances, will immediately differentiate the surgically amenable problem from the nonsurgical respiratory distress syndrome (hyaline membrane disease) and the aspiration pneumonias.

In summary, the symptoms of respiratory distress are (a) restlessness, (b) tachypnea, (c) retractions, and (d) cyanosis. Work-up includes (a) history, (b) physical examination, (c) chest x-ray, (d) evaluating arterial blood gases, and (e) passing a nasogastric catheter with a radiopaque marker.

PROBLEM 1

FINDINGS

1. There is a history of sudden onset of respiratory distress at any time in the newborn period. These symptoms may be intermittent or progressively worsening.
2. Examination reveals that the heart sounds loudest in one hemithorax (usually the right) and a suggestion of unequal movement of hemithoraces. The abdomen is scaphoid. There are decreased breath sounds in one hemithorax (usually the left). All of these signs may be minimal.
3. Chest x-ray shows a bowel pattern in one hemithorax. There is a mediastinal shift with compression of the contralateral lung. The diaphragm may be markedly elevated or indistinct. Abdominal bowel gas is sparse or absent (Fig. 22).
4. The nasogastric catheter reaches the stomach, but the stomach may be in an abnormal position.
5. Arterial blood gases indicate respiratory acidosis and hypoxia.

DIAGNOSIS

The diagnosis is diaphragmatic hernia (Bochdalek).

DIFFERENTIAL DIAGNOSIS

Differential diagnosis includes eventration of the diaphragm and congenital cystic adenomatoid degeneration of the lung.

MANAGEMENT

1. Institute immediate and continuous nasogastric decompression to avoid further bowel distention and consequent progressive respiratory embarrassment.
2. Provide respiratory support as needed and achieve venous and arterial cannulation for resuscitation, acid–base corrections, and monitoring.

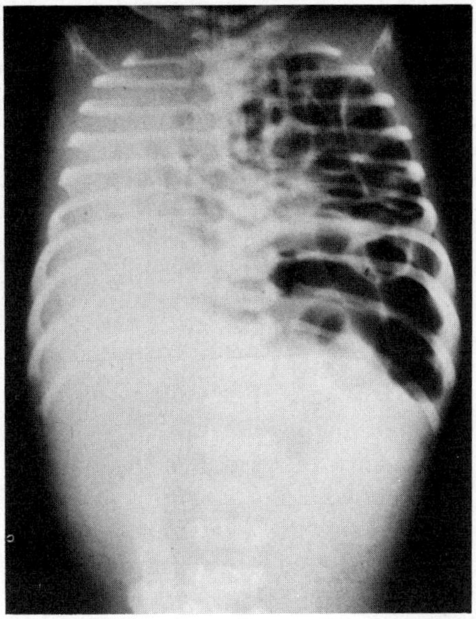

FIG. 22. Radiograph of newborn with left diaphragmatic hernia (Bochdalek). Note mediastinum shifted to the right, bowel gas pattern in left chest, and sparcity of bowel gas in abdomen.

3. Maintain careful attention to temperature control during evaluation and resuscitation.
4. Perform corrective surgery as soon as adequate resuscitation is accomplished.

DISCUSSION

The baby who is symptomatic from diaphragmatic hernia within the first 8 hours has a markedly different prognosis from the child who is asymptomatic until after 24 hours.[4-7] Eventration of a hemidiaphragm is rarely symptomatic in the first 24 hours of life and may be overlooked for weeks or many months[8] (see Figs. 35 and 36). Congenital cystic lung disease, when localized enough to be confused with diaphragmatic hernia, is rarely symptomatic so early in life.[9] Since these two entities present later and with less acute symptoms, a more thorough investigation, including contrast studies of the gastrointestinal tract, is warranted to avoid misdiagnosis.[10,11] The child in trouble from diaphragmatic hernia early in life frequently combines both ventilatory insufficiency from lung compression with perfusion insufficiency from decreased venous return to the heart caused by the mediastinal shift. These babies require rapid resuscitation, correction of acidosis, and emergency surgery.[4] Occasionally, thoracic decompression becomes an integral factor in resuscitation itself. In large series from competent institutions,[5,6] this lesion carries a prohibitive mortality which can only be improved by diagnosis from the earliest symptoms, very rapid resuscitation, and early surgery before a severe ventilatory perfusion insult occurs.

Endotracheal intubation should be avoided during resuscitation if possible. It should certainly not be done routinely, because of the high risk of developing a pneumothorax, which is rapid in onset and progressive secondary to traumatic bronchopleural fistula. If pneumothorax develops or is already present, a chest tube should be inserted prior to surgery. This may be needed on either or both sides, for either side may develop a pneumothorax spontaneously or secondary to assisted ventilation. If a baby is improved and stabilized and then suddenly his respiratory function worsens again, pneumothorax is the most probable cause. Notwithstanding this relative caution against endotracheal intubation, ventilation by bag and mask is absolutely contraindicated, for this pushes air directly into the bowel.

Because of the interference with perfusion and cardiac output, cellular injury may occur, resulting in marked extravascular fluid shifts. Resuscitation must therefore include volume maintenance, but fluid overload must also be diligently avoided.

FACTORS IMPORTANT IN POSTOPERATIVE MANAGEMENT

1. Ventilatory support should be given as needed.

2. Continued volume support may be very important, particularly if the infant was hypoperfused preoperatively. Use of albumin-containing balanced salt solutions will provide increased intravascular oncotic pressure, helping to offset the tendency toward extravascular fluid shifts, which may produce interstitial pulmonary edema.[12,13] Cautious judgment is required in the use of albumin, however, for it may prove to be deleterious if pulmonary capillary integrity is impaired.[14]

3. The lung on the herniated side is often compressed or hypoplastic. Attempts to expand it rapidly by mechanical positive-pressure ventilation or high-pressure chest tube suction will rupture the lung, with resultant pneumothorax. If mechanical ventilation is required, consideration should be given to bilateral chest tube drainage for prophylactic decompression. A balanced underwater system is required.[15]

4. Even with the transthoracic approach, several days of postoperative intravenous fluid, electrolyte, and nutritional support may be necessary until intestinal function resumes.

5. When these infants have trouble postoperatively, it is usually the result of preoperative hypoventilation and hypoperfusion resulting in severe interstitial pulmonary edema and generalized hypoxic tissue damage.[16,17] Marked

intrapulmonary shunting occurs, and arterial oxygen tensions fall precipitously. Respiratory acidosis becomes uncontrollable, and "reopening" of the ductus arteriosus may ensue, further shunting blood from the pulmonary circuit. It is this combination of events that produces the frequent mortality in these infants.

Recent thinking about these patients has been directed toward finding the etiology of the postoperative severe pulmonary insufficiency. For a long time, this was blamed on hypoplastic lungs, but in fact most of these children have a perfectly adequate lung on the side opposite the hernia. Frequently, immediately postoperatively, the lung is able to function well. Most can achieve PO_2 levels of over 100 mm Hg and some well over 300 mm Hg. However, a relentlessly downhill course then ensues, eventually with severe intractable hypoxia and death.

The pathophysiology may be related to the fact that the severe compression of the lung prevents development of interstitial edema. However, ischemic damage has occurred. Once the hernia is repaired and the compression released, the edema develops and oxygenation is inhibited. This would explain the frequent excellent oxygenation immediately after repair, as well as the very rapid deterioration.

Present therapy is directed toward increasing inspired oxygen concentrations and positive-pressure breathing. When preoperative ischemia has been minimal, this frequently suffices and the lungs improve in a few days.

In more severely injured patients, however, even high-pressure breathing and 100 percent inspired oxygen levels may fail to oxygenate the child adequately. One reason for this failure may be due to hypertension in the pulmonary circuit, either in the hypoplastic ipsilateral lung alone, or in both lungs. Investigations are being directed toward pharmacologically reducing the pulmonary hypertension.[4] Also of interest is the question of whether gross shunting through either the ductus arteriosus or the foramen ovale or both as a result of the pulmonary hypertension is contributing to the hypoxemia.[4]

PROBLEM 2

FINDINGS

1. There is a history of progressive respiratory distress.
2. Examination may show "dextrocardia." The abdomen appears to be normal.

3. Chest x-ray shows a hyperinflated lobe (usually left upper). Frequently, the picture is confused with pneumothorax. The mediastinum may be shifted, but the diaphragm is clearly present; it may be flattened. The intra-abdominal intestinal gas pattern is normal. The hyperaerated area is large but localized: ie, it does not radiate out symmetrically from the hilum.
4. The nasogastric catheter is in the stomach, which is in normal position.

DIAGNOSIS

The diagnosis is lobar emphysema.

DIFFERENTIAL DIAGNOSIS

The differential diagnosis is congenital cystic adenomatoid degeneration of the lung.

MANAGEMENT

1. Provide careful, continuous monitoring by clinical observation, serial blood gases, and frequent chest films.
2. Perform lobectomy when needed for rapidly progressive or persistent impairment of respiratory function.
3. Continue nasogastric decompression to minimize abdominal distention.

DISCUSSION

Occasionally, more than one lobe or side may be involved. The respiratory impairment may be insidiously progressive. Emergency lobectomy may be required.[9,18] Confusion with pneumothorax may lead to a tube thoracostomy, which may worsen symptoms by creating tension pneumothorax. If symptoms are not severe or progressive, the process may stabilize and lobectomy may be avoided. An associated lesion is cystic lung disease or congenital cystic adenomatoid degeneration of the lung, in which numerous hyperinflated cysts are seen on x-ray and may be confused with the appearance of bowel-in-the chest of diaphragmatic hernia[11,19] (Fig. 23). The presence of a normal abdominal bowel gas pattern helps in differentiating them. Lateral chest x-rays and upper gastrointestinal series may be helpful. Pulmonary scanning has proved to be useful in diagnosing lobar emphysema.[20]

POSTOPERATIVE MANAGEMENT

1. Continue ventilatory support as needed.
2. Hypovolemia is rarely a significant problem.
3. Thoracotomy tubes can be managed in routine fashion (unlike those in diaphragmatic hernia, which require a balanced system).

PROBLEM 3

FINDINGS

1. There is a history of sudden onset and progressive symptoms of respiratory distress.
2. Examination reveals decreased breath sounds over one side of the chest. "Dextrocardia" is not apparent. The abdomen appears to be normal.

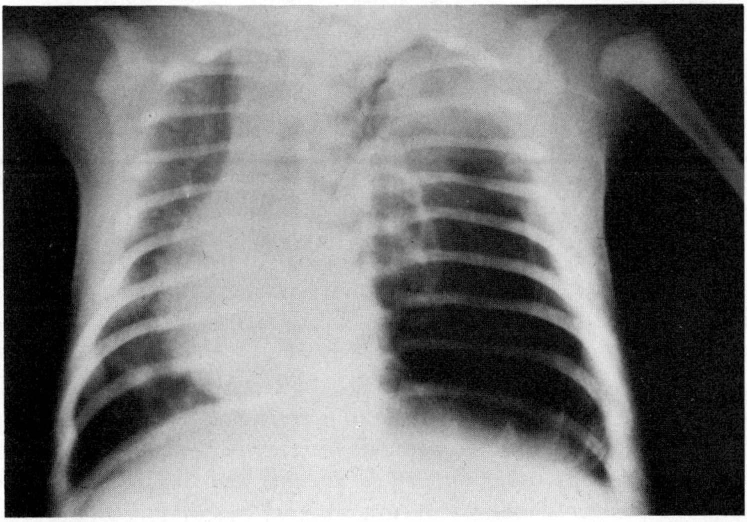

FIG. 23. Chest radiograph of infant with congenital cystic adenomatoid degeneration of lung. Note diffuse involvement of lung and confusing "diaphragm-like" appearance of left interlobar fissure with "bowel-loop" pattern in left lower lung field.

3. Chest x-ray shows pneumothorax and various degrees of lung collapse. The collapse is always symmetrical toward the hilum. Mediastinal shift may or may not be present. Lateral chest x-ray may show prominent mediastinal air (between sternum and heart). Intestinal gas pattern is normal.
4. The nasogastric tube is in a normally positioned stomach.
5. Arterial blood gases usually indicate mild respiratory acidosis unless severe collapse is already present, in which case they confirm severe respiratory insufficiency.

DIAGNOSIS

The diagnosis is pneumothorax.

MANAGEMENT

1. Rapid judgments are needed to decide whether tension pneumothorax with contralateral lung compression and interference with venous return is developing.
2. Frequent and continuous observations for development of tension must be made.
3. On the basis of points 1 and 2, decide whether to apply (a) oxygen therapy and observe, (b) needle aspiration, or (c) tube thoracostomy.

DISCUSSION

Spontaneous development without apparent underlying etiology is common.[21] Pneumothorax frequently follows endotracheal resuscitation.[22] Underlying etiologies such as eventration, diaphragmatic hernia, emphysema, and hyaline membrane disease can usually be ruled out by the chest x-ray. Prolonged chest tube thoracostomy with high-vacuum suction may be required. However, in the absence of an underlying pathologic entity, surgery is seldom indicated. Associated anomalies are rare.

With the increasing use of endotracheal tubes and positive-pressure ventilation in the resuscitation of tiny infants with respiratory distress, forced entry of air into extra-alveolar spaces is becoming a common complication. Rupture of an alveolus allows air to dissect into the perivascular tissue planes and exit into the pleural space or the mediastinum, resulting in pneumomediastinum or pneumothorax. An even more serious problem is pneumopericardium with tamponade. The supposed explanation for the alveolar rupture is forceful entry of air into a partially obstructed alveolus (air block syndrome).[23]

TREATMENT

Pneumomediastinum requires no treatment. Pneumothorax is treated as outlined above. Pneumopericardium requires urgent decompression of the pericardial sac if the infant is to survive.

POSTOPERATIVE MANAGEMENT

Continued effective functioning of the chest tube must be ensured by frequent clinical observation and chest x-rays. Additional tubes may be needed when large leaks from the lung tissue are present (Fig. 24).

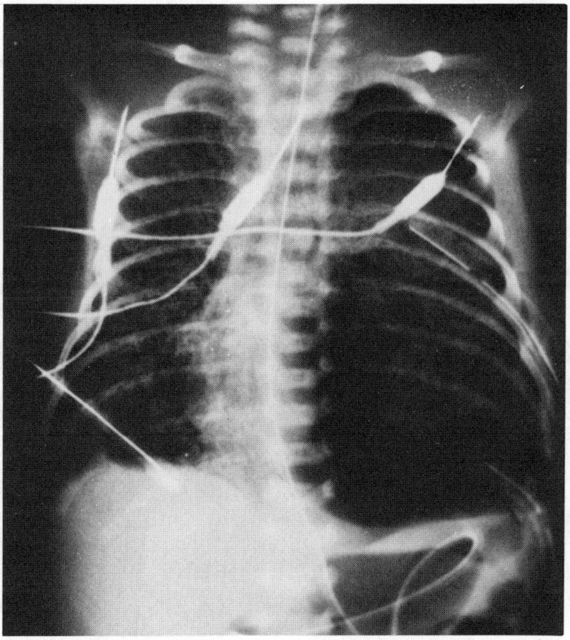

FIG. 24. Infant with pneumothorax. Persistent left pneumothorax despite presence of two thoracostomy tubes.

PROBLEM 4

FINDINGS

1. History reveals, in addition to respiratory distress and cyanosis, excessive nasopharyngeal saliva. Early feedings are followed by non-bile-stained vomiting. Maternal hydramnios may have been present.
2. Examination reveals a normal-appearing baby who is usually less than 2500 g and is often somewhat premature. Early chest auscultation is normal. The abdomen may show progressive distention.
3. Chest x-ray shows a wide, air-filled pouch in the neck or upper mediastinum. Aspiration pneumonia may be noted, usually in the right upper lobe. The nasogastric tube, if in place, will be seen to stop at the end of the pouch at about T_3 (Fig. 25). Visible parts of the abdomen frequently show hyperaeration of the intestines.

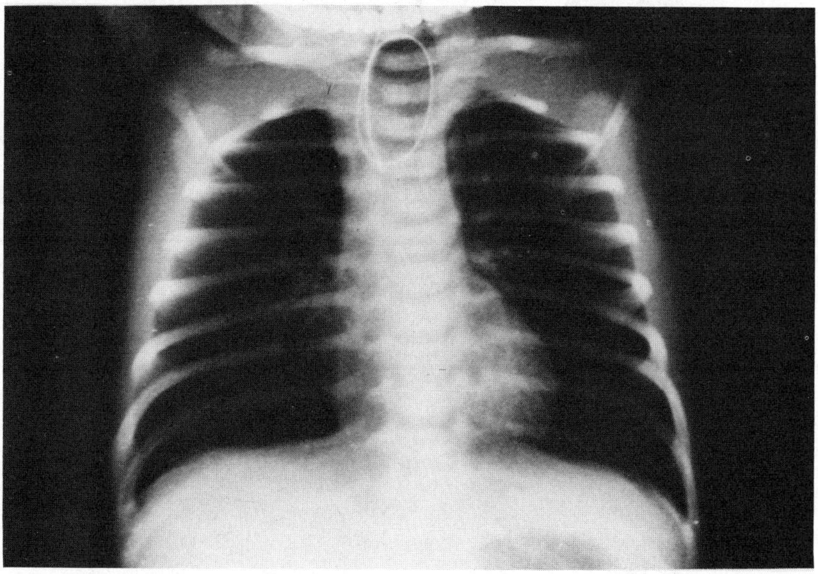

FIG. 25. Infant with esophageal atresia. Radiopaque tube is coiled in blind pouch in superior mediastinum. Note gastric air confirming the presence of a typical fistula from the trachea to the distal esophageal segment.

4. The nasogastric tube, as noted, meets obstruction at about 12 cm and fails to reach the stomach. Too small a tube may enter the trachea, pass through the tracheoesophageal fistula, and reach the stomach, confusing interpretation.[24] Use of at least a 12 French tube will avoid this confusion.

DIAGNOSIS

The diagnosis is esophageal atresia with or without tracheoesophageal fistula.

MANAGEMENT

1. Position infant with head elevated 45 degress and prone as much as possible to minimize the chance of aspiration.
2. Place a sump catheter in the blind proximal pouch and connect it to constant suction. The Replogle Tube*(a 10 French sump catheter) was specifically designed for this purpose.[25]
3. Provide additional oral or nasal pharyngeal suctioning of saliva as needed.
4. Because maintenance of the erect–prone position is so important, accompany the baby to x-ray.
5. Rapid evaluation and early decisions about surgery are urgent (see discussion).

DISCUSSION

Positioning the baby as described is essential to prevent aspiration pneumonia. Two sources must be considered. The first, regurgitation of oral contents from the blind proximal pouch, is avoided by constant sump suctioning. The second, and more significant source, is regurgitation of acid gastric juice up the distal esophagus and through the fistula. Proper positioning helps to minimize this. The prone position makes regurgitation from the anterior stomach to the posteriorly placed esophagus more difficult, while ascension in the esophagus is limited by the 45 degree head-up factor (Fig. 26).

Most textbooks suggest contrast studies of the upper pouch to confirm the diagnosis.[26,27] These are rarely necessary, however, and add a high risk of

*Replogle Tube, Argyle, Sherwood Medical Industries, St. Louis, Mo.

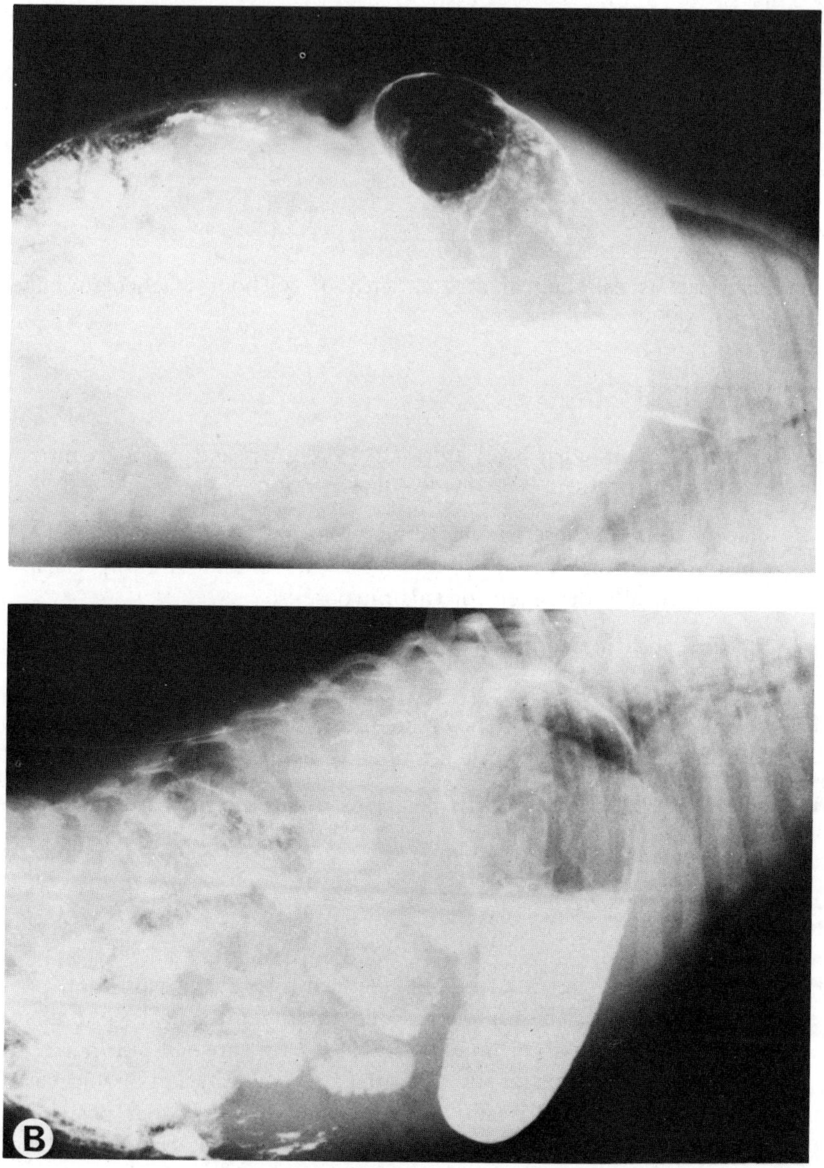

FIG. 26. Radiographs of supine child showing: A. *Contrast material pooling in dorsum of stomach and refluxing easily into esophagus.* B. *In the prone, head-elevated position dye pools in anterior stomach away from esophagus, helping to prevent reflux and aspiration of gastric contents through tracheoesophageal fistula. (Radiographs courtesy of Dr. Dale Johnson)*

aspiration of the contrast material[28] (see Fig. 8). The responsible surgeon should do them, of course, if the diagnosis is unclear or the possibility of a rare esophageal stenosis amenable to simple dilatation exists. Water-soluble contrast agents should be avoided, as their high osmolality damages the respiratory epithelium if aspirated. Barium is the best choice if one must be used.

About 90 percent of esophageal atresias are as described above: a blind proximal pouch with the distal esophagus entering the tracheobronchial tree as a fistula. Approximately 8 percent are pure esophageal atresia with no fistula.[29] Here the risk of gastric aspiration is not present. Tube decompression of the the proximal pouch suffices until gastrostomy and cervical esophagostomy can be performed electively under local anesthesia. Usually, a colon interposition is required to bridge the atretic gap and can best be done after the child is 6 months of age.[30] Recent investigations by Hendren into the use of dual magnetic bougies placed in the proximal and distal esophageal pouches and intermittently coapted by an electromagnetic field[31] may eliminate the need for interposition procedures with their considerable morbidity.

Tracheoesophageal Fistula without Atresia

The pure tracheoesophageal fistula or so-called H type is even more rare. Diagnosis of this entity is difficult but should be suspected when repeated aspiration pneumonias, abdominal distention, and/or a history of coughing with feedings is present.[32] Diagnosis by bronchoscopy with the infant bronchoscope with optical telescope* is the quickest and safest method.[33] Transcervical ligation of the fistula provides easy treatment, but delayed diagnosis makes the mortality from this lesion significant.[32] Any child who presents symptoms of coughing with feedings with or without cyanosis should have early bronchoscopy. Older methods, requiring tracheal and esophageal intubations with dye injections and x-ray studies, are less productive and more hazardous. Bronchoscopy without specialized newborn instruments is often not definitive.[32]

Laryngotracheoesophageal Cleft

A rare lesion that must be considered in a child with aspiration pneumonia and feeding-related ventilatory difficulties is laryngotracheoesophageal cleft. This lesion varies from a short segment extending from larynx to crycoid all the way to one in which total cleft of the airway to the bronchial level leaves the esophagus and trachea as a single tube.[34,35] Early recognition of the lesion and definition of its extent are essential to survival. Bronchoscopy with specialized pediatric optical endoscopes should be performed urgently when the diagnosis is suspected.

*Karl Storz Endoscopy-America, Los Angeles, Calif.

Associated Lesions

Congenital heart disease is associated with esophageal atresia in as high as 20 percent of cases. Over half of the lesions are serious.[36] Anorectal atresias and other intestinal atresias are seldom seen but occur more frequently than by random association. Duodenal atresia not infrequently accompanies esophageal atresia, especially the pure atresia without tracheoesophageal fistula variety. When it accompanies the more common form with tracheoesophageal fistula, gastrostomy becomes even more urgent, because the forced entry of air into the stomach through the fistula may overexpand the stomach and rupture it (Fig. 27). The gastric dilatation also increases the risk of regurgitation of gastric contents into the tracheobronchial tree. Anesthetic management of these babies must be very well thought out to prevent either of the above complications.

When the baby has been a suitable candidate for primary repair of the esophagus and fistula, we have performed gastrostomy, decompressing the stomach, repaired the duodenal atresia, and then proceeded to thorocotomy.

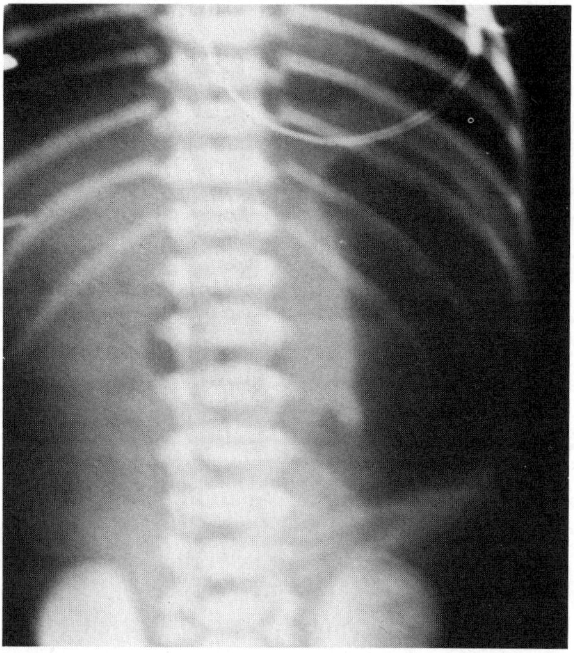

FIG. 27. Abdominal radiograph of infant with esophageal atresia and tracheoesophageal fistula showing obstruction in duodenum. Both duodenal atresia and malrotation were found at exploration.

Gastrostomy is the only urgent procedure, however, and could be performed under local anesthesia in a sick baby.

Finally, imperforate anus is associated with either duodenal or esophageal atresia at a greater than random incidence.

TREATMENT

Surgical intervention is urgent in the esophageal atresia associated with tracheoesophageal fistula. The choice of procedure depends on the clinical condition of the baby. Emergency primary repair should be done only when the following criteria are satisfied: (a) Normal chest to auscultation and chest x-ray, (b) no obvious unevaluated cardiac abnormalities, (c) PO_2 of 60 mm Hg or higher in room air, and (d) knowledgeable anesthetic and ventilatory support personnel available.

Prematurity, low birth weight, and other anomalies (rectal, intestinal) are not contraindications to primary repair as previously thought.[37-39] The slightest evidence of pneumonia or other respiratory insufficiency is a contraindication, however.

If primary repair cannot be accomplished as an urgent procedure, emergency gastrostomy under local anesthesia is mandatory, to decompress the intestines and offset the risk of gastric regurgitation and continued soilage of the tracheobronchial tree. The upper pouch sump catheter and the head-up position should be maintained during the procedure.

Once the diagnosis of pneumonia is made, it must be treated continuously and vigorously until all of the above criteria are met, regardless of how long this requires (average, 10 to 14 days). Under these circumstances a central venous line for TPN is indicated to support the infant's nutritional state over the two to three weeks of intestinal inanition. Feedings should not be attempted through the gastrostomy tube as long as the fistula remains open, because reflux with entry of gastric contents into the tracheobronchial tree cannot be avoided. Daily endotracheal intubation for tracheobronchial lavage and suction may hasten clearing of the pneumonia. Ultrasonic nebulization adds an important therapeutic modality in thinning secretions and thereby allowing them to be cleared more easily.[40] The hazard of water intoxication caused by absorption of large amounts of water through the respiratory epithelium[41] can be prevented by adjustments in administration of intravenous fluids.

When significant improvement in the pneumonia has been delayed due to difficulty in clearing secretions, we have not hesitated to perform tracheostomy. This greatly improves secretion-clearing ability, which is hampered by the weakened valsalva ability of the infant with the tracheoesophageal fistula. The fistula prevents the baby from achieving adequate coughing pressure.

PRINCIPLES OF POSTOPERATIVE MANAGEMENT

1. Ultrasonic nebulization is mandatory. Maintenance fluids must almost always be reduced by 30 to 40 percent to allow for the high bronchiolar membrane absorption when ultrasonic mist is used.[40,41]

2. Nasal and oral pharyngeal suctioning should be performed at least hourly with a catheter marked at 10 cm to prevent it from reaching the anastomosis. The catheter should be used to stimulate the infant to cough.

3. Twice daily endotracheal intubation and lavage of the tracheobronchial tree with intravenous quality saline solution by a knowledgeable and skilled physician is needed in an occasional infant for adequate clearing of secretions but should be minimized. When the above criteria for surgery are adhered to and postoperative ultrasonic mist is used, this intubation is rarely required.

4. Keep the neck flexed (neutral position). Never hyperextend it, as this levers the anastomotic site of the esophagus across the vertebral column, leading to anastomotic dehiscence.

5. In other respects postoperative positioning is less important than it is preoperatively. Once the baby begins oral feedings, however, it is important to keep him sitting up. Esophageal reflux is a very common problem in these infants and may lead to aspiration pneumonia.[42,43] The reflux usually subsides with time.

6. Culture the tracheal aspirate daily and change antibiotics appropriately.

7. Use endotracheal ventilatory support as needed. When indicated, tracheostomy may be life-saving.

8. Monitor blood gases.

9. Maintain the chest drainage tube (usually an extrapleural tube) and withhold oral and gastrostomy feedings until the integrity of the anastomosis is established unequivocally by barium swallow at five to six days postoperatively. Continue parenteral alimentation if available during this period.

10. Other anomalies may be corrected at any time.

11. Maintain surveillance for associated cardiac anomalies, especially during the second week of life.

Obviously the esophageal atresias may present with signs of gastrointestinal obstruction rather than, or in addition to, respiratory distress. In fact, if every child who shows any increase of or difficulty with saliva were immediately studied by nasogastric intubation with a radiopaque 12 French catheter followed by a portable chest x-ray, respiratory distress might be eliminated as a presenting symptom complex of esophageal atresia. As mentioned previously, the mothers of many of these infants have hydramnios. The obstetrician could suspect the diagnosis even before the pediatrician sees the child and could initiate the investigation with a tube and an x-ray.

PROBLEM 5

FINDINGS

1. History shows an otherwise normal-appearing child presenting early in the neonatal period with noisy breathing, restlessness, opisthotonic posturing, and moderate to severe retractions. Cyanotic spells may follow. Changes in position, especially placing the baby prone, may improve respirations.
2. Examination may reveal nothing abnormal, or it may show a small recessed chin. There may be a high arched palate or an actual cleft. Retractions of the intercostal muscles and nasal flaring are obvious.
3. Chest x-ray is almost invariably normal unless the child has aspirated.
4. The nasogastric tube may not pass through the nose. Otherwise it reaches the stomach without difficulty and is seen in proper position on the x-ray.
5. Arterial blood gases will reflect the severity of obstruction. Unless the baby is cyanotic, PO_2 is often adequate, but PCO_2 may reflect the ventilatory impairment, approaching 60 mm Hg.

DIAGNOSIS

The diagnosis is congenital airway obstruction.

DIFFERENTIAL DIAGNOSIS

Differential diagnosis includes choanal atresia, Pierre Robin syndrome, laryngomalacia, hypopharyngeal tumors, subglottic cysts, laryngotracheal hemangiomas and lymphangiomas, tracheomalacia, and vascular arch anomalies (rings).

MANAGEMENT

The severity of airway obstruction that the child is having will dictate the urgency of the resuscitative efforts, but too often these lesions are treated too nonchalantly. Airway obstruction is a potentially rapidly lethal entity. Early thorough evaluation is therefore mandatory.

Arterial blood gases will confirm the clinical impression that the baby is working to breathe. If a rising PCO_2 indicates fatigue with impending ventilatory failure, immediate, thorough investigation should be carried out.

If the nasogastric tube will not pass through the nares, choanal atresia may be present. This is a very rare lesion, however. An oral airway should then completely relieve the obstruction. If it does not, the diagnosis of choanal atresia should be doubted, and further evaluation of the total airway should be completed.

Evaluation of the ease with which the infant can be intubated is a most important factor in planning further work-up. If this can be easily accomplished, further studies can then be obtained with greater security. Therefore, after adequately oxygenating the child and suctioning secretions, a gentle awake larygoscopy should be performed. This will allow identification of palatal defects, hypopharyngeal tumors, subglottic masses, and, usually, laryngomalacia.

In no lesions are identified at laryngoscopy and if intubation can be easily accomplished if needed, lateral neck films may then be obtained to evaluate the airway. The baby should be accompanied to the radiology area by someone who can manage his airway capably and who has the needed equipment with him.

If endotracheal intubation appears to be difficult or if, after the lateral airway films, no supraglottic cause for the obstruction has been found, the child should be transported to the operating room, where awake intubation and general anesthesia should be carried out.

Thorough evaluation of the airway should then be performed starting with a good view of the hypopharynx and epiglottis, progressing to the larynx and cords, and then completing tracheobronchial evaluation using an optical telescopic infant bronchoscope.*

The infant should then be reintubated and allowed to awaken thoroughly. If no major obstructive lesion has been found, the infant may be extubated and observed carefully. Reintubation or tracheostomy may be required, depending on the specific findings and the ventilatory function of the baby after extubation.

DISCUSSION

If choanal atresia is confirmed, the baby must be guaranteed a stable oral airway or else should be intubated until surgical correction of the atresia is achieved. Newborns are obligate nose breathers, so this is a lethal lesion.[44]

The micrognathia of the Pierre Robin syndrome is usually obvious. Cleft palate is not universally present.[45] It is thought that the mechanical disadvantage of the tongue-protrusion muscles due to the short mandible allows

*Karl Storz Endoscopy-America, Inc., Los Angeles, Calif.

the tongue to become lodged in the posterior pharynx, occluding the epiglottis. With swallowing, the infant then creates a vacuum in the esophagus, sealing the hypopharynx with the tongue.

Often all that is needed is to suspend a nasopharyngeal tube in place to prevent the vacuum seal from forming.[46,47] Previous attempts to hold the tongue forward with wires or the Beverly Douglas tongue–lip adhesion were variably successful.[48] Tracheostomy is the most dependable means of ensuring a patent airway, but should rarely be needed.

Tumors are usually benign and may be cysts, hemangiomas, or lymphangiomas. If they can be easily removed acutely, tracheostomy can be avoided, but modern tracheostomy techniques make this procedure highly acceptable. Ill-conceived and poorly timed operative procedures should not be attempted as a means of avoiding tracheostomy.

The epiglottis may be the key to the whole problem. Often the only abnormality found is an "omega"-shaped, floppy epiglottis which seems capable of causing the stridor. If no other lesion is present and the baby shows no evidence of ventilatory decompensation, nothing need be done. Eventually, maturation of the epiglottis and larynx will alleviate the symptoms.

The trachea should be observed through the bronchoscope while the baby is breathing spontaneously. It may appear more ovoid in shape and tend to collapse with inspiration. This tracheomalacia is unusual, and the diagnosis is probably made too frequently.

Vascular arch ring anomalies may be noted as areas of extrinsic compression during bronchoscopy but are probably best diagnosed by subsequent barium swallow and arteriography.

FACTORS OF IMPORTANCE IN POSTOPERATIVE MANAGEMENT

Regardless of the lesion found or the procedure required, attentive nursing care in an intensive care setting is mandatory until airway stability is ensured.

OTHER ANOMALIES PRESENTING WITH RESPIRATORY DISTRESS

Rare thoracic lesions such as cysts, mediastinal tumors (lymphangiomas and teratomas), and rare diaphragmatic hernias (foramen of Morgagni and paraesophageal) may present as respiratory distress in the newborn but are much less common than the entities discussed above.

CHAPTER 2

CONGENITAL ANOMALIES THAT PRESENT WITH GASTROINTESTINAL OBSTRUCTIVE SYMPTOMS

The symptoms of gastrointestinal obstruction include vomiting and distention, increased salivation, and failure to defecate.

GASTROINTESTINAL OBSTRUCTION

The majority of surgical emergencies of the newborn present with one or more of these symptoms. Some may also be the earliest signs of sepsis, congenital heart disease, and a variety of nonsurgical metabolic or digestive abnormalities.

A rapid and logical evaluation should be instituted to sort out the entities that are amenable to surgical correction. The presence of a mechanically obstructing lesion must be assumed until it is totally ruled out. Only such an attitude will bring about early diagnosis and treatment and thereby achieve improved survival from these lesions. There is no greater tragedy than the loss of an otherwise normal child from a lesion that earlier surgery could have corrected. To discuss thoroughly the presenting symptoms, evaluate the findings, and outline the special work-up required for each lesion that commonly presents with vomiting and distention would require not a chapter, but a sizable part of a textbook of pediatric surgery. It is the purpose of this section to give an overview of the subject and provide the physician with a logical course to pursue. Additional entities are outlined in Section III.

DISCUSSION

Vomiting suggests obstruction. It is this that must be established or ruled out. The character of the vomitus often gives some clue to the level of obstruction. Preduodenal blockage results in non-bile-stained vomiting. Postpyloric obstruction usually produces bile in the vomitus. It is a cardinal rule of pediatrics that *green vomitus, no matter how small the amount, is a surgical emergency until proved not to be so*. Disregard for this rule has cost many a baby his life.

Our first principle, then, is that *vomiting, especially bile-stained vomiting, suggests mechanical obstruction*, and the work-up must be directed toward rapidly establishing the presence of obstruction or ruling it out.

The baby who vomits non-bile-stained material without distention probably has esophageal atresia, achalasia, diaphragmatic hernia, sepsis, or a nonobstructive lesion. Pyloric and duodenal obstructions present with upper abdominal distention. All lesions beyond the ligament of Treitz usually produce generalized abdominal distention.

Although every obstructive lesion requires prompt recognition and rapid decompression with thoughtful and intelligent management of dehydration, electrolyte imbalance, hypoglycemia, and accompanying physiologic upsets, only four of the obstructive entities require emergency surgery to ensure survival. These are esophageal atresia, malrotation, free gastrointestinal perforations, and Hirschsprung's disease. Esophageal atresia is discussed in Chapter 1 of this section. Because of their frequency and importance, malrotation, perforation, and Hirschsprung's disease are emphasized here.

MALROTATION

Gastrointestinal obstruction between the pylorus and ligament of Treitz must be considered malrotation until completely ruled out. This is our second important principle.

Often it is impossible to rule out malrotation without surgery. Malrotation produces not only obstruction of the duodenum, complete or incomplete, but also strangulation of the superior mesenteric artery from volvulus of the small bowel mesentery. Thus, the entire small intestine is at risk. Only early recognition and prompt surgical correction can salvage the infant. Recognition of the entity can be difficult. The following principles may be helpful:

1. Any obstruction developing after continuity of the gastrointestinal tract has been demonstrated by x-ray or the rectal passage of gas or transitional stools must be considered malrotation and volvulus. This is our third rule: *Once a child has demonstrated intestinal continuity, he must never be considered to have intestinal discontinuity on a congenital atresia basis again*.

2. Duodenal obstruction should always suggest malrotation. Only an ab-

solutely classical "double-bubble" film of duodenal atresia with complete obstruction and no evidence of prior passage of gas beyond this point should allow surgery to be delayed. Even when these criteria are completely satisfied, malrotation is only relatively and not absolutely ruled out. Here a barium enema may give added support.[49] Delay in treatment is warranted only when the baby's condition makes anesthesia as great a risk as is missing the diagnosis of malrotation.

3. Partial duodenal obstructions with air beyond the duodenum may be caused by annular pancreas and partial intrinsic duodenal webs. However, these should be treated by emergency surgery, because malrotation as the obstructing cause can never be completely ruled out unless the upper gastrointestinal series shows an unequivocally normal C loop of the duodenum and clearly left-sided ligament of Treitz.

4. Usually an upper gastrointestinal contrast x-ray study will demonstrate duodenal obstruction and failure of the duodenal C loop to cross back to the

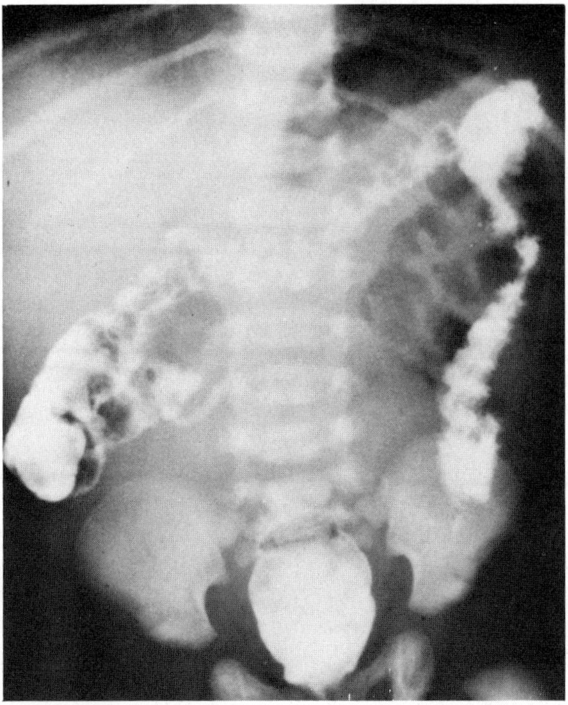

FIG. 28. Barium contrast enema study illustrating possible confusion in identifying cecum. Cecum is actually folded back on itself and points, along with appendix, toward the umbilicus. The patient had a malrotation.

left upper quadrant when malrotation is present.[49,50] Barium enema demonstrates the cecum in the right upper quadrant but does not show the duodenal obstruction. Barium enema may be confusing because the cecum may move about freely and appear to be normally located in the right lower abdomen[49] (Fig. 28). In the face of obstructive symptoms, if either study is abnormal, surgery should be performed urgently. If the first study done appears to be normal, the other should be done.

5. Malrotation with strangulating volvulus may present as in utero obstruction of the duodenum, in which case no gas will have passed the duodenum, and obvious confusion with duodenal atresia will result. If in doubt, a good, safe rule is to operate at once.

FREE PERFORATIONS OF THE GASTROINTESTINAL TRACT

The diagnosis of free perforation of an intestinal viscus should be suspected when sudden, rapid distention of the abdomen occurs with or without emesis. Physical findings reveal a tympanitic abdomen with absence of liver dullness, a sign that should always be sought in a distended infant.

Although an erect, plain abdominal film is almost always diagnostic, showing free air beneath the diaphragms (Fig. 29), it is more important to be able to recognize the presence of free air on the supine abdominal film, as this is more frequently obtained. This will show a decreased right upper quadrant liver opacity with a hazy air bubble over the liver, an outlining by air of the falciform ligament as it crosses to the liver substance,[51] and thickening between the loops of bowel suggesting peritonitis. Often, there is a ghost-like appearance to the bowel loops as air outlines the outside of the walls (Fig. 30).

In the past, the usual sites of perforation in the neonatal period were the stomach, the cecum, and the duodenum.[52-54] Etiologies varied, were often obscure, and were frequently related to distal obstruction. Early recognition and prompt surgical correction salvaged some of these infants before overwhelming sepsis became irreversible.

Modern, up-to-date neonatal units have markedly improved the survival of small premature babies with hyaline membrane disease and aspiration pneumonias. As a result, all such units have experienced a marked increase in neonatal necrotizing enterocolitis (NEC), which usually presents first radiographically with air in the bowel wall (pneumatosis intestinalis) and pneumobilia (actually pylephlebitis with air in the portal venous system from

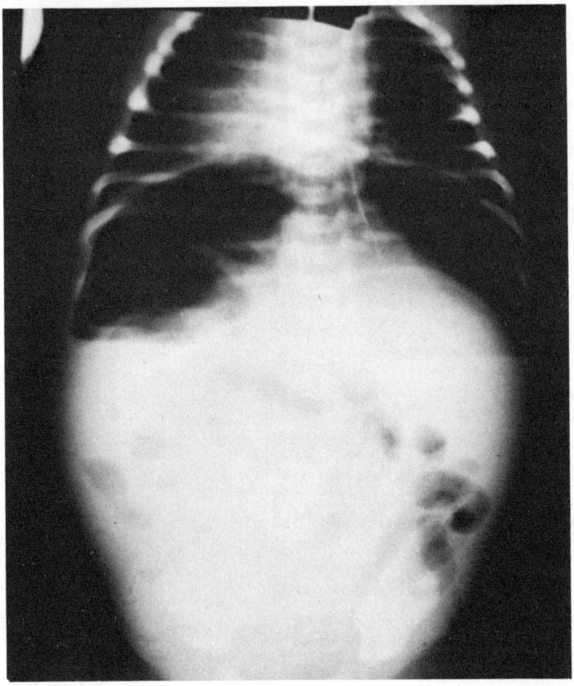

FIG. 29. Upright abdominal radiograph showing extensive intraperitoneal air in a patient with a gastrointestinal perforation.

gas-forming gram-negative organisms).[55,56] Unfortunately, a common sequel to these signs is intestinal perforation with leakage of air and intestinal contents into the peritoneal cavity. This entity is now overwhelmingly the most common cause of neonatal bowel perforation.

Its etiology remains obscure, but it is thought to be due to ischemic injury to the intestine from mesenteric vasoconstriction. This results from the infant's excessive reaction to stresses such as hypoxia, hypovolemia, and hypothermia. Figure 5 illustrates the mechanism of this low-flow state. Barlow and her associates at Babies' Hospital, New York, have shown that NEC can be produced in laboratory rats by a combination of severe hypoxic stress (near agonal asphyxiation) and formula feeding.[57] The fact that rat breast milk protects the stressed rats from developing NEC has led them and other investigators to propose that the infantile immune deficiency combines with the ischemic injury to allow invasion of the bowel wall by enteric organisms. After colonizing the bowel wall, these organisms spread to the liver through the portal venous system and then produce systemic bacteremia and endotoxemia.

Outline of Proposed Mechanism of Necrotizing Enterocolitis (after Barlow)[57]

1. There is ischemic stress to infant.
2. Reactive mesenteric vasoconstriction occurs.
3. Mucosal ischemic injury reduces barrier to invasion by enteric bacteria.
4. Immune deficiency of newborn allows rapid colonization and spread of organisms.
5. Injured bowel wall becomes gangrenous and perforates with further septic challenge.

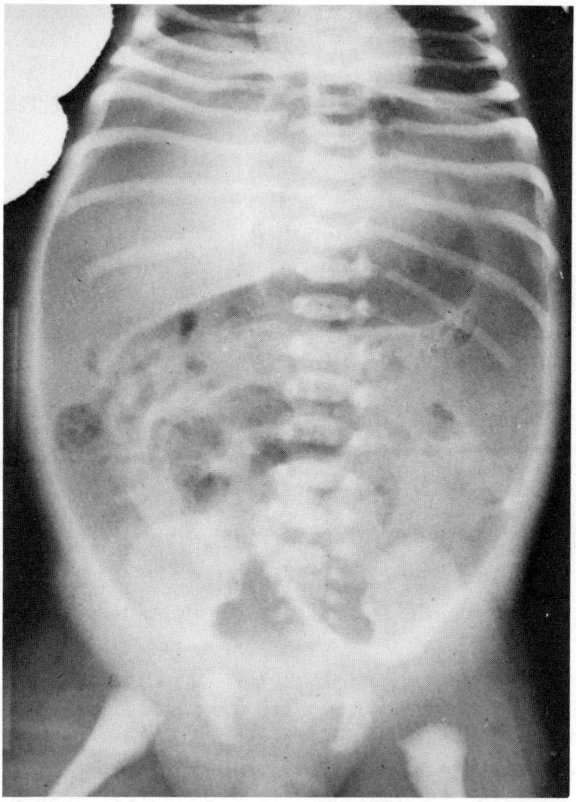

FIG. 30. Radiograph of infant with massive free air in the peritoneal cavity. The falciform ligament is clearly outlined. The normal liver opacity is absent from the right upper quadrant. The entire abdomen appears as a large gas bubble.

It has been further hypothesized that breast milk provides immune factors to the rat, accounting for its protective effect.[57] Human breast milk has not seemed to be as consistently protective for human infants, but valid data have been difficult to acquire.

Inability to handle hyperosmolar loads in an immature gastrointestinal tract leading to reflex vasospasm and mesenteric vascular insufficiency has also been considered a causative or important contributing factor.

TREATMENT

Once necrotizing enterocolitis has resulted in free perforation of the bowel, surgical treatment is mandatory (Fig. 31). The infant should be prepared with rapid volume expansion with blood, albumin, and Ringer's lactate. Massive doses of antibiotics with good broad-spectrum and gram-negative effectiveness should be given.

The choice between local resection of the perforation with primary intestinal reconstitution or resection with enterostomy and later reconstruction depends on the extent of bowel involvement and the surgeon's evaluation of the integrity of the surrounding intestine. The lesions may be localized to a short segment of distal ileum or cecum, may destroy the entire intraperitoneal colon, or less commonly may involve the entire bowel extensively.

Time spent mechanically cleaning the spilled contents from the peritoneal cavity is probably worthwhile, as it eliminates sites for bacteria to flourish in poorly vascularized substrate. Despite heroic surgical efforts, the mortality after perforation remains high.[58,59] Therefore, earlier recognition of necrotizing enterocolitis with vigorous treatment directed toward preventing perforation should be the goal of all who deal with these infants.[58-60]

The early symptoms of NEC are abdominal distention; loose, seedy stools frequently positive for occult blood or streaked with blood; and bile-stained emesis or gastric aspirate. Signs of sepsis such as apnea, bradycardia, and hypothermia may occur concomitantly, especially in more premature infants.

Abdominal films taken at this point may clearly demonstrate air in the bowel wall or may show only an ileus-type picture with a "bubbly" or "dirty" appearance to the intraluminal contents. Contrast enema studies are contraindicated because of the risk of perforation.

If complete bowel rest with nasogastric decompression, massive parenteral antibiotic therapy, and full fluid, electrolyte, and indicated transfusion therapy is instituted at this point, most infants will improve rapidly. Ventilatory and myocardial assistance should be provided as needed along with requisite thermal maintenance. Bowel rest will be required for at least three weeks, or recrudescence rates will be significant. Therefore, central venous TPN should be instituted after the acute septic phase is controlled.

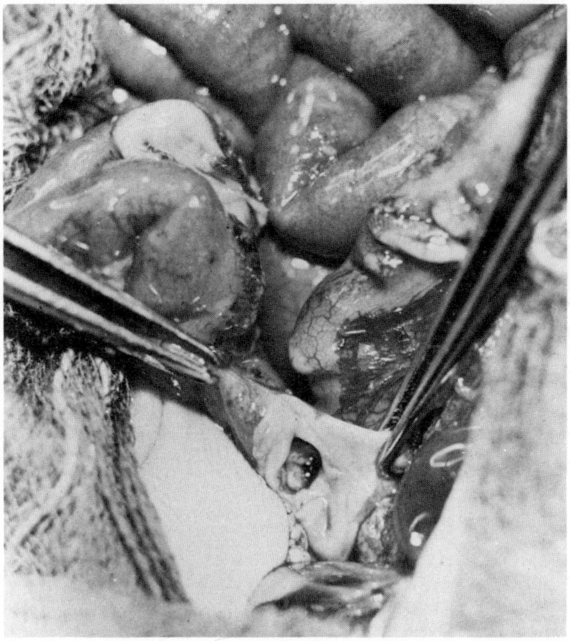

FIG. 31. Necrotizing enterocolitis with area of bowel necrosis and large perforation. Other loops of intestine are dilated, thickened, and hyperemic.

Careful, frequent reevaluation of the infant in the 24 to 48 hours after onset of the disease will identify the baby who is failing to respond to medical treatment. Survival rates are better when surgical intervention is provided prior to frank perforation.[58,59]

Our indications for surgery, other than for evidence of free perforation, are the following:

1. Development of signs of peritonitis: tenderness with significant guarding, edema of the abdominal wall, or hyperemia of the abdominal wall
2. Failure to stabilize in 12 hours after instituting treatment, ie, persistent bradycardia, apnea, and hypothermia
3. Development of sepsis after therapy has been instituted
4. Palpation of a mass representing an insidious walled-off perforation or gangrenous bowel without free intraperitoneal air

When infants are operated on for the above indications, necrotic bowel with impending perforation is usually found. Although peritonitis exists and bowel organisms can be cultured from the peritoneal fluid, ,the absence of gross contamination with bowel contents seems to allow treatment to overcome the septic insult more often than when actual gross spillage has occurred.

When postoperative sepsis progresses to disseminated intravascular coagulopathy, multiple exchange transfusions will restore the clotting mechanism and raise and stabilize the platelet count.[61] Severe toxicity can be reversed when this course of therapy is pursued vigorously. We have also utilized prophylactic exchange transfusion when sepsis has been anticipated. Our results with this technique have been very good, but random studies to demonstrate statistical significance have not been done.

HIRSCHSPRUNG'S DISEASE (AGANGLIONIC MEGACOLON)

The third of the entities requiring emergency surgery in the newborn period is aganglionic megacolon. The urgency relates to the presence or imminent development of pseudomembranous enterocolitis with its attendant high mortality. This is another lesion that must be thought of and suspected in order to make the diagnosis. In the usual case the child is distended, may vomit, has usually passed some meconium, and may have even passed transitional or milk stools. He may have diarrhea, and, when enterocolitis supervenes, a tan, foul-smelling liquid diarrhea is common. The entity should be suspected whenever a baby presents with obstruction far down the intestinal tract. Any baby failing to pass meconium in 24 hours should be a suspect.[3] Differential diagnosis includes meconium ileus, ileal atresia, colonic atresia, and meconium plug syndrome. Contrast enema studies will go far in differentiating among these. Barium should be used only if Hirschsprung's disease is the prime suspect. For the others, high-osmolar, water-soluble contrast agents will often be curative as well as diagnostic.[62,63]

Except for abdominal distention, physical examination in Hirschsprung's disease is normal. The idea that a normal rectal exam rules it out is falacious. Hirschsprung's disease is a functional, not an anatomic, obstruction.

If the barium enema is not diagnostic and the symptoms persist, rectal biopsy should be done. However, a colostomy must be done urgently and should not be delayed pending rectal biopsy if enterocolitis is present.

The child who fails to pass meconium in the first 24 hours of life and becomes distended, later to pass a meconium plug after contrast enema, should remain suspect of having aganglionic megacolon even though he continues to stool. Babies of diabetic mothers frequently have a meconium plug syndrome[64,65] or small left colon syndrome.[66,67] All other babies with this syndrome should be evaluated thoroughly for Hirschsprung's disease. If after relief of the meconium plug the baby seems to function normally, a barium enema should be repeated at 1 month of age. When this principle has been ignored, insidious obstruction, enterocolitis, and free perforation have resulted.

NEWBORN OBSTRUCTIVE ENTITIES AND ORGANIZED PLAN OF SORTING OUT THE DIAGNOSIS

Newborn obstructive entities include the following:

1. Esophageal atresia with tracheoesophageal fistula
2. Esophageal atresia without fistula
3. Achalasia
4. Pyloric atresia
5. Pyloric stenosis
6. Duodenal atresia
7. Duodenal stenosis
8. Annular pancreas
9. Malrotation with volvulus
10. Jejunal atresia
11. Ileal atresia
12. Meconium ileus
13. Colonic atresia
14. Colonic stenosis
15. Aganglionic megacolon
16. Meconium plug syndrome; small left colon syndrome
17. Gastrointestinal perforation

18. Meconium peritonitis (in utero perforation)
19. Imperforate anus
20. Cloacal anomalies

Question: Can some orderly approach be found to identify the diagnosis rapidly from this long list of entities presenting in or near the newborn period, all of which present with symptoms of gastrointestinal obstruction?

Answer: Yes. An organized approach to data gathering as outlined below will differentiate these lesions most of the time.

HISTORY

Hydramnios suggests complete obstruction above the midjejunum. This is the level where swallowed amniotic fluid is resorbed and subsequently excreted back to the pool through the fetal urinary tract. Therefore, the presence of hydramnios suggests a high gastrointestinal obstruction such as esophageal, duodenal, or proximal jejunal atresia.[2]

PHYSICAL FINDINGS

The child who is born distended probably has meconium ileus (cystic fibrosis), hydrometrocolpos with rectovaginal fistula (cloacal anomaly), or meconium peritonitis. Rapid onset of distention suggests abnormal air entry into the gut, as in tracheoesophageal fistula. Non-bile-stained vomiting suggests obstruction above the entry of the bile duct into the duodenum. Imperforate anus is obvious most of the time. Rectal atresia with open anus is a very rare lesion. Careful inspection of the perineum will reveal the presence of cloacal anomalies such as hydrometrocolpos with rectovaginal fistula.

Thus, from history and examination we can diagnose imperforate anus and hydrometrocolpos and can suspect a high obstruction if hydramnios was present. The character of the vomitus will help to suggest the obstructive level, and immediate or early distention will point toward certain entities.

Next pass a good-sized radiopaque nasogastric tube until it stops. Aspirate the "stomach" until empty and note the quantity and color of the aspirate. Inject 50 ml of air and clamp the tube. Obtain flat and upright x-rays that include the neck, chest, abdomen, and pelvis simultaneously (babygram).

If bile is present in the aspirate, the tube has reached the stomach, and obstruction beyond the bile duct should be suspected. If the tube has stopped in the upper mediastinum, esophageal atresia is diagnosed. If air is present in the stomach and intestines, a tracheoesophageal fistula accompanies the atresia of the esophagus.

Pyloric atresia is extremely rare. Pyloric stenosis rarely presents before 2 weeks of age, and is an incomplete obstruction. Achalasia rarely presents in the first few days, is most often confused with pyloric stenosis, and no radiographic evidence of obstruction is present.

Next note the gas pattern in the intestines. Do not err in thinking that much time is required to establish a normal gas pattern. Remember that with the first breath taken by the baby air enters the stomach. The duodenum is reached with the second or third. Within an hour air should have progressed well along the small bowel, reaching the cecum by 6 hours at the latest. Most of the colon should be filled by 8 to 12 hours.

Air is an excellent contrast agent in the newborn. Within 1 to 2 hours after birth a definite decision about the presence of obstruction can be made, and its level (high or low) estimated.

If the duodenum is completely or partially obstructed and the vomitus or aspirate is green, differentiate among duodenal atresia, duodenal stenosis, annular pancreas, and malrotation. Operate immediately if the latter cannot be totally ruled out (see the section on malrotation).

Further perusal of the plain x-rays will reveal intra-abdominal calcifications if meconium peritonitis is present. A triad of findings suggestive of meconium ileus includes disparity in the size of the distended loops, a mottled or "soapy" appearance to the intraluminal contents, and sparse or absent air–fluid levels in the distended loops on the upright film. Free air will usually be clearly seen on the upright film when perforation has occurred. When present immediately after birth, it usually is accompanied by meconium peritonitis or is the result of gastric rupture from resuscitation by bag and mask. When perforation presents later (two to five days), NEC or Hirschsprung's disease must be considered.

When the blockage appears to be in the mid-small bowel, atresia of the jejunum or ileum is the usual cause. Since malrotation with volvulus and strangulation of the mesentery is probably a major in utero etiology for those atresias, the risk of further volvulus and strangulation of the blood supply to the remaining bowel makes operative investigation urgent.

If duodenal obstruction is present and there is any reason to delay surgery, upper gastrointestinal contrast evaluation with barium should be done to completely rule out malrotation if possible.

If the obstruction is at the distal ileal or colonic level by plain x-rays, contrast enema should now be done. Unless air in the rectum clearly demonstrates that the colon is patent, high-osmolar, water-soluble material should be the initially chosen agent. It will prevent barium impaction and usually will be therapeutic for meconium ileus, meconium plug syndrome, or small left colon syndrome. A dependable intravenous line should be established, and balanced salt solution should be administered to offset the fluid losses into the gut caused by the highly osmolar contrast material.[68]

When the study reveals small-caliber "unused" colon, the diagnoses to be considered are meconium ileus, ileal atresia, a very long segment meconium plug, small left colon syndrome, or Hirschsprung's disease involving the entire colon. The latter is rare.

If the triad of plain film findings suggesting meconium ileus is present and the colon appears small and "beady" with inspissated mucus, attempts to reflux the enema into the ileum should be made and, if successful, repeated until good clearing of the ileum with extensive small bowel reflux is achieved. If nothing has suggested meconium ileus, the colon is unused but not "beady," and reflux fails, ileal atresia is the probable diagnosis. Meconium plugs will be seen and will evacuate with the enema. Small left colon syndrome is essentially indistinguishable from meconium plug except for involving the bowel higher up. They are probably variations of the same entity. Hirschsprung's disease of the usual shorter segment variety will show the caliber change to a more dilated proximal bowel. Remember the caution that meconium plug syndrome and small left colon syndrome be investigated subsequently to rule out underlying aganglionosis. Finally, congenital colonic atresias and stenoses are very rare and will be obvious from the contrast enema.

The point made previously in this section that, once a baby has demonstrated a patent gastrointestinal tract, congenital atresias are forever ruled out should be kept in mind. The infant who is initially well and demonstrates an open, functioning gastrointestinal tract and then becomes ill with vomiting and distention will most likely have either necrotizing enterocolitis or malrotation with volvulus.

The above presents an organized program for information accrual that will allow rapid differentiation of what otherwise may seem to be an overwhelming list of possibilities. Adherence to this program will enable even the totally inexperienced physician to diagnose a major obstructive congenital anomaly within the first few hours of life and provide referral for proper treatment before complications threaten the baby's survival.

CHAPTER 3

CONGENITAL ANOMALIES THAT PRESENT AS AN ABDOMINAL MASS

INTRODUCTION

Abdominal masses in the newborn period are unusual findings but should be easily noted on physical examination, since the newborn's abdomen is so easy to palpate. The location, mobility, and characteristics of the mass determine the subsequent course of investigations. A highly mobile intra-abdominal mass is probably a duplication or a mesenteric cyst. Most masses are retroperitoneal flank masses and are relatively immobile. Differentiation among benign anomalies of the urinary tract and malignant tumors of renal, hepatic, or neural ganglionic or adrenal origin can best be achieved by planning sophisticated evaluations after thorough study of the intravenous pyelogram. Table 1 presents the salient features of the various lesions. The following points of expansion of the table are cogent:

1. Wilms' tumor is a renal lesion. Therefore, distortion of the calyces with some residual function is the usual pattern (Fig. 32). Large-sized tumors may cross the midline, but calcification is unusual. When present it is coarse and easily seen on x-ray. Hypertension may be present, possibly from renal artery stenosis. In the newborn period, renal tumors are usually the more benign mesoblastic variant.[69] Pulmonary metastases are highly unusual.

2. Abdominal neuroblastoma, on the other hand, is usually (but not always) extrarenal, and thus it displaces the kidney from its usual site (Fig. 33). Distortion is less prominent. This tumor frequently crosses the midline. Fine, speckled calcifications are common but are usually not discernible by routine x-ray studies. Hypertension is common and may be accompanied by sweating, flushing, and diarrhea.

TABLE 1: PHYSICAL AND RADIOLOGIC CHARACTERISTICS OF ABDOMINAL MASSES

Diagnosis	Location	Accompanying Signs and Symptoms	Character Mobility	Calcification Transillumination	IVP	UGI	Special Studies
Mesenteric cyst	Variable	Occasional emesis	Soft, cystic Highly mobile	No Yes	Normal	Occasional partial obstruction	Sonogram
Gastrointestinal duplications	Variable	Occasional intestinal obstruction or intussusception	Smooth, firm Moderate to highly	No Rarely	Normal	Occasional partial obstruction	Sonogram
Choledochal cyst	RUQ	Jaundice	Small, smooth, firm None	No No	Normal	Extrinsic duodenal distortion	Liver scan, liver function studies sonogram
Wilms' tumor	Flank	Fever, hypertension	Solid, smooth Minimal	Occasionally No	Distorted calcyes	Mass effect	Chest x-ray, IV cavagram, bone marrow
Neuroblastoma	Flank, occasionally midline or pelvic	Pain, fever, hypertension debility	Solid, irregular Minimal	Occasionally No	Displaced calcyes	Mass effect	Chest x-ray, IV Cavagram, bone survey, bone marrow, VMA*
Hepatic tumors	RUQ	Occasionally ascites	Smooth,hard None	Occasionally No	Usually normal	Occasional gastric or duodenal displacement	Liver function studies, ateriography
Multicystic kidney or hydronephrosis	Flank	Rare	Solid, smooth Moderate	None Yes	Usually nonfunction	Occasional mass effect	Sonogram
Hydrometrocolpos	Midabdomen and/or pelvic area	Perineal anomalies, peritonitis	Smooth Minimal	No No	Bilateral hydronephrosis, displaced hydroureters	Bowel displaced to upper abdomen	Urogenital sinogram, IVP

*VMA, Vanillyl Mandilic Acid

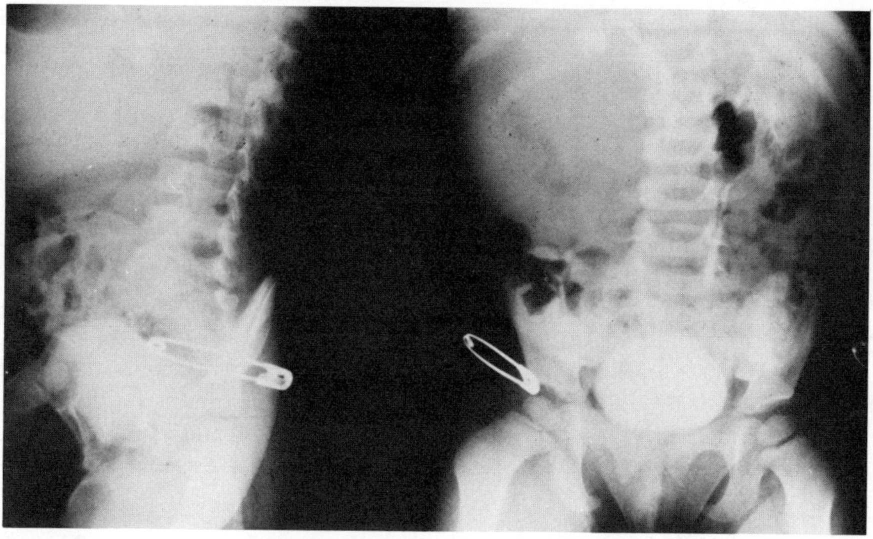

FIG.32 Intravenous pyelogram of infant with Wilms' tumor showing distortion of calyceal pattern.

FIG.33. Intravenous pyelogram of 7-week-old infant with right suprarenal neuroblastoma. The kidney is rotated and displaced, but the calyceal pattern is maintained.

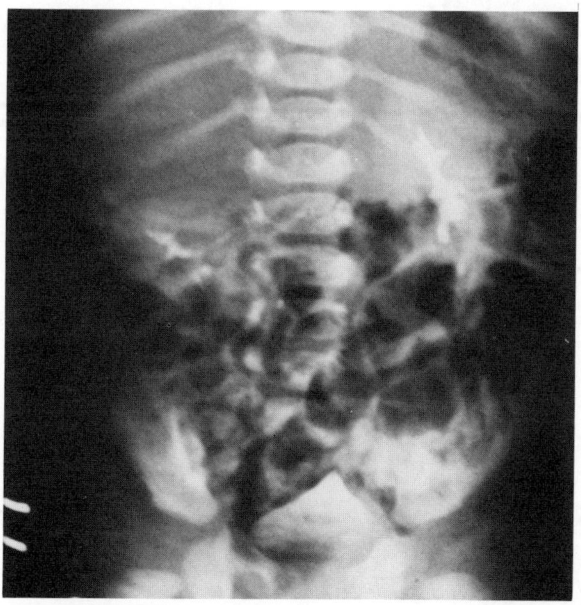

3. Multicystic kidney is either a dysplastic kidney or the extreme result of ureteral obstruction or atresia. Usually there is nonfunction on the intravenous pyelogram on the involved side.

4. Note that only the intra-abdominal cysts and intestinal duplications are highly mobile. The first sign of a duplication may be obstruction, frequently due to intussusception of the duplication.

5. Hepatic tumors are rarely accompanied by jaundice, whereas choledochal cysts almost invariably are.

6. Unless a fairly certain diagnosis of a flank mass can be made preoperatively from the intravenous pyelogram, the preoperative special studies should include those for both neuroblastoma and Wilms' tumor.

7. Retrograde pyelograms are unnecessary and probably contraindicated because pressure or manipulation may rupture a Wilms' tumor. If differentiation from obstructive uropathy is impossible from the intravenous study, cautious retrograde studies by a urologist with extensive experience with infants is permissible.

CHAPTER 4

CONGENITAL ANOMALIES THAT PRESENT AS OBVIOUS DEFORMITIES

The following anomalies are easily recognizable at birth and require no special diagnostic tests. Since each is discussed in detail in Section III, they will not be discussed here individually.

1. Imperforate anus
2. Hydrometrocolpos with imperforate anus
3. Gastroschisis
4. Omphalocele
5. Exstrophy of the bladder
6. Urachal remnants
7. Omphalomesenteric duct remnants
8. Cleft lip; cleft palate
9. Cystic hygroma
10. Meningomyelocele
11. Sacrococcygeal teratoma
12. Hernias; hydroceles
13. Undescended testicles

CHAPTER 5

BLEEDING IN THE NEWBORN PERIOD

For practical purposes, massive gastrointestinal bleeding, especially bloody vomitus, in the neonatal period is not a surgical problem. An exact etiology is rarely established.[70]

There are certain essential steps to take, the first of which is to determine by the Apt test[71] whether the blood is maternal (swallowed) or fetal in origin. To be accurate, this test must be done on the blood from the center of a clot.

The platelet count, prothrombin time, and partial thromboplastin time must be determined to rule out intrinsic clotting-factor deficiencies.[72] Serial hematocrits are sine qua non to demonstrate actual blood loss and evaluate continued bleeding. Blood pressure monitoring will help define severe shock. Appropriate blood must be obtained for transfusion, and blood loss replaced when necessary after bleeding and clotting studies have been obtained.

A large indwelling venous catheter must be in place at all times. A large nasogastric tube for iced saline irrigations should be placed.

Most neonatal hemorrhage stops spontaneously and does not recur. Persistence of bleeding should, of course, be followed by a thorough gastrointestinal evaluation. A surgically amenable lesion is rarely found.[70,73] Presently, the one exception to this is necrotizing enterocolitis, which frequently presents with extensive rectal hemorrhage. In the modern neonatal unit, blood in the stool should be investigated immediately to rule out NEC.

The passage of blood or bloody stool in a distended baby with green gastric aspirates or emesis may also indicate the presence of necrosing bowel from malrotation and strangulating volvulus. Urgent evaluation is mandatory.

REFERENCES

1. Moore KL: The Developing Human. Clinically Oriented Embryology. Philadelphia, Saunders, 1973, pp 97, 172
2. Lloyd JR, Clatworthy HW, Jr: Hydramnios as an aid to the early diagnosis of congenital obstruction of the alimentary tract. A study of the maternal and fetal factors. Pediatrics 21:903, 1958
3. Swenson O, Sherman JO, Fisher JH: Diagnosis of congenital megacolon: an analysis of 501 patients. J Pediatr Surg 8:587, 1973
4. Dibbins AW, Weiner ES: Mortality from neonatal diaphragmatic hernia. J Pediatr Surg 9:653, 1974
5. Johnson DG, Deaner RM, Koop CE: Diaphragmatic hernia in infancy: factors affecting the mortality rate. Surgery 62:1082, 1967
6. Snyder WH, Jr, Greaney EM: Congenital diaphragmatic hernia: 77 consecutive cases. Surgery 57:576, 1965
7. McNamara JJ, Eraklis AJ, Gross RE: Congenital posterolateral diaphragmatic hernia in the newborn. J Thorac Cardiovas Surg 55:55, 1968
8. Bishop HC, Koop CE: Acquired eventration of the diaphragm in infancy. Pediatrics 22:1088, 1958
9. Crawford TJ, Cahill JJ: The surgical treatment of pulmonary cystic disorders in infancy and childhood. J Pediatr Surg 6:251, 1971
10. Avnet NL: Roentgenologic features of congenital bilateral anterior diaphragmatic eventration. Am J Roentgenol Radium Ther Nucl Med 88:743, 1962
11. Buntan WJ, Isaacs H, Jr, Payne VC, Jr, et al: Lobar emphysema, cystic adenomatoid malformation, pulmonary sequestration, and bronchogenic cyst in infancy and childhood: a clinical group. J Pediatr Surg 9:85, 1974
12. Moss GS, Siegel DC, Cochin, et al: Effects of saline and colloid solutions on pulmonary function in hemorrhagic shock. Surg Gynecol Obstet 133:53, 1971
13. Moylan FMB, O'Connell KC, Todres ID, et al: Edema of the pulmonary interstitium in infants and children. Pediatrics 55:783, 1975
14. Holcroft JW, Trunkey DD: Pulmonary extravasation of albumin during and after hemorrhagic shock in baboons. J Surg Res 18:91, 1975
15. Padula RT: Postoperative management. In Sabiston DC, Jr, Spencer FC (eds): Gibbon's Surgery of the Chest. Philadelphia, Saunders, 1976. pp 176, 177
16. Raphaely RC, Downes JJ, Jr: Congenital diaphragmatic hernia: prediction of survival. J Pediatr Surg 8:815, 1973
17. Boix-Ochoa J, Peguero G, Seijo G, et al: Acid–base balance and blood gases in prognosis and therapy of congenital diaphragmatic hernia. J Pediatr Surg 9:49, 1974
18. Kennedy JH, Rothmann BF: The surgical treatment of congenital lobar emphysema. Surgery 121:253, 1965
19. Monclair T, Schistad G: Congenital pulmonary cysts versus a differential diagnosis in the newborn: diaphragmatic hernia. J Pediatr Surg 9:417, 1974

20. Mauney FM, Jr, Sabiston DC, Jr: The role of pulmonary scanning in the diagnosis of congenital lobar emphysema. Am Surg 36:20, 1970
21. Srouji MN: Pneumothorax and pneumomediastinum in the first three days of life. J Pediatr Surg 2:410, 1967
22. Chernick V, Reed MH: Pneumothorax and chylothorax in the neonatal period. J Pediatr 76:624, 1970
23. Mansfield PB, Graham CB, Beckwith JB, et al: Pneumopericardium and pneumomediastinum in infants and children. J Pediatr Surg 8:691, 1973
24. Gwinn JL, Lee FA, Crowe CC, et al: Radiologic case of the month. Am J Dis Child 126:621, 1973
25. Replogle RL: Esophageal atresia—plastic sump catheter for drainage of the proximal pouch. Surgery 54:296, 1963
26. Mustard WT, Ravitch MM, Snyder WH, Jr,et al (eds): Pediatric Surgery. Chicago, Year Book, 1969
27. Randolph JG: Congenital anomalies of the esophagus. In Sabiston DC, Jr, Spencer FC (eds): Gibbon's Surgery of the Chest. Philadelphia, Saunders, 1976
28. Koop CE, Hamilton JP: Atresia of the esophagus: factors affecting survival in 249 cases. Z Kinderchir 5:319, 1968
29. Holder TM, Cloud DT, Lewis JE, Jr, et al: Esophageal atresia and tracheoesophageal fistula. A survey of its members by the Surgical Section of the American Academy of Pediatrics. Pediatrics 34:542, 1964
30. Waterston DJ: Reconstruction of the esophagus. In Mustard WT, Ravitch MM, Snyder WH, Jr, et al (eds): Pediatric Surgery, Chicago, Year Book, 1969, p 400
31. Hendren WH, Hale JR: Esophageal atresia treated by electromagnetic bougienage and subsequent repair. J Pediatr Surg 11:713, 1976
32. Bedard P, Girvan DP, Shandling B: Congenital H-type tracheoesophageal fistula. J Pediatr Surg 9:663, 1974
33. Gans SL, Berci G: Inside tracheoesophageal fistula: new endoscopic approaches. J Pediatr Surg 8:205, 1973
34. Pettersson G: Inhibited separation of larynx and the upper part of trachea from oesophagus in a newborn. Acta Chir Scand 110:250, 1955
35. Novoselac M, Dangel P, Fisch U: Laryngotracheoesophageal cleft. J Pediatr Surg 8:963, 1973
36. Haight C: Congenital esophageal atresia and tracheoesophageal fistula. In Mustard WT, Ravitch MM, Snyder WH, Jr, et al (eds): Pediatric Surgery. Chicago, Year Book, 1969, p 358
37. Abrahamson J, Shandling B: Esophageal atresia in the underweight baby: a challenge. J Pediatr Surg 7:608, 1972
38. Koop CE, Hamilton JP: Atresia of the esophagus: increased survival with staged procedures in the poor risk infant. Ann Surg 162:389, 1965
39. Holder TM, McDonald VG, Jr, Woolley MM: The premature or critically ill infant with esophageal atresia: increased success with a staged approach. J Thorac Cardiovasc Surg 44:344, 1962
40. Swenson O, Grana L, Hausam T: Use of ultrasonic nebulizer during anesthesia. J Pediatr Surg 6:554, 1971
41. Edmunds LH, Jr, Downes JJ: Assisted ventilation in infants. In Sabiston DC, Jr, Spencer FC (eds): Gibbon's Surgery of the Chest. Philadelphia, Saunders, 1976

42. Ashcraft KW, Goodwin C, Amoury RA, et al: Early recognition and aggressive treatment of gastroesophageal reflux following repair of esophageal atresia. J Pediatr Surg 12:317, 1977
43. Pieretti R, Shandling B, Stephens CA: Resistant esophageal stenosis associated with reflux and repair of esophageal atresia: a therapeutic approach. J Pediatr Surg 9:355, 1974
44. Francesoni G: The nose. In Mustarde JC (ed): Plastic Surgery in Infancy and Childhood. Philadelphia, Saunders, 1971, p 261
45. Matthews DN: Hare lip and cleft palate. In Mustarde JC (eds): Plastic Surgery in Infancy and Childhood. Philadelphia, Saunders, 1971, p 1
46. Stern LM, Fonkalsrud EW, Hassakis P, et al: Management of Pierre Robin syndrome in infancy by prolonged nasoesophageal intubation. Am J Dis Child 124:78, 1972.
47. Fletcher MM, Blum SL, Blanchard CL: Pierre Robin syndrome. Pathophysiology of obstructive episodes. Laryngoscope 79:547, 1969
48. Lindsay WK: Lips, tongue, and floor of the mouth. In Mustarde JC (ed): Plastic Surgery in Infancy and Childhood. Philadelphia, Saunders, 1971, p 122
49. Simpson AJ, Leonidas JC, Krasna IH, et al: Roentgen diagnosis of midgut malrotation. Value of upper gastrointestinal radiographic study. J Pediatr Surg 7:243, 1972
50. Berdon WE, Baker DH, Bull S, et al: Midgut malrotation and volvulus: which films are most helpful. Radiology 96:375, 1970
51. Miller RE: Perforated viscus: a new radiological sign. Radiology 74:65, 1960
52. Tucker AS, Izant RJ, Jr: How serious are gastrointestinal perforations in infancy? Radiology 81:112, 1963
53. Lloyd JR, Benson CO: Gastrointestinal perforations in the newborn. In Mustard WT, Ravitch MM, Snyder WH, Jr, et al (eds): Pediatric Surgery. Chicago, Year Book, 1969, p 797
54. Mustard WT, Ravitch MM, Snyder WH, Jr, et al: Pediatric Surgery. Chicago, Year Book, 1969
55. Wolfe JN, Evans WA: Gas in portal veins of the liver in infants: a roentgenographic demonstration with post mortem anatomical correlation. Am J Roentgenol Radium Ther Nucl Med 74:486, 1955
56. Touloukian RJ, Berdon WE, Amoury RA, et al: Surgical experience with necrotizing enterocolitis in the infant. J Pediatr Surg 2:389, 1967
57. Barlow B, Santulli T, Heird WC, et al: An experimental study of acute neonatal enterocolitis—the importance of breast milk. J Pediatr Surg 9:587, 1974.
58. Stevenson JK, Oliver TK, Jr, Graham B, et al: Aggressive treatment of neonatal necrotizing enterocolitis. J Pediatr Surg 6:28, 1971
59. Dudgeon DL, Coran AG, Lauppe FA, et al: Surgical management of acute necrotizing enterocolitis in infancy. J Pediatr Surg 8:607, 1973
60. Bell MJ, Kosloske AM, Benton C, et al: Neonatal necrotizing enterocolitis: prevention of perforation. J Pediatr Surg 8:601, 1973
61. Gross S, Melhorn D: Exchange transfusion with citrated whole blood for disseminated intravascular coagulation. J Pediatr 78:415, 1971
62. Noblett HR: Treament of uncomplicated meconium ileus by Gastrografin enema: a preliminary report. J Pediatr Surg 4:190, 1969
63. Wagget J, Bishop HC, Koop CE: Experience with Gastrografin enema in the treatment of meconium ileus. J Pediatr Surg 5:649, 1970

64. Clatworthy HW, Howard WHR, Lloyd J: The meconium plug syndrome. Surgery 39:131, 1956
65. Ellis DG, Clatworthy HW, Jr: The meconium plug syndrome revisited. J Pediatr Surg 1:54, 1966
66. Davis WS, Campbell JB: Neonatal small left colon syndrome. Am J Dis Child 129:1024, 1975
67. Philippart AI, Reed JO, Georgeson KE: Neonatal small left colon syndrome: intramural not intraluminal obstruction. J Pediatr Surg 10:733, 1975
68. Rowe MI, Seagram G, Weinberger M: Gastrografin induced hypertonicity: the pathogenesis of a neonatal hazard. Am J Surg 125:185, 1973
69. Bolande RP, Brough AJ, Izant RJ, Jr: Congenital mesoblastic nephroma in infancy. Pediatrics 40:272, 1967
70. Sherman NJ, Clatworthy HW, Jr: Gastrointestinal bleeding in neonates: a study of 94 cases. Surgery 62:614, 1967
71. Apt L, Downey W, Jr: Melena neonatorum: the swallowed blood syndrome. J Pediatr 47:6, 1955
72. Glader BE, Buchanan GR: The bleeding neonate. Pediatrics 58:548, 1976
73. Koop CE: Gastrointestinal bleeding in infants and children. In Blakemoore WS, Ferguson LK (eds): Current Perspectives in Gastroenterology. New York, Harper, 1967

SECTION 3

MANAGEMENT OUTLINE OF COMMON PEDIATRIC SURGICAL PROBLEMS

INTRODUCTION

The first two sections of this book were designed to provide a background of knowledge about the general care of the newborn infant and to facilitate the diagnostic evaluation of the infant from the presenting symptoms. The purpose of adding this third section is to provide a quick reference outline of the overall management of the most common entities seen in pediatric surgery. It should be viewed as an overall "sketch" of each problem, designed to help get the care program underway and to provide direction for the long-range plan.

It is repetitious of some of the entities discussed in Section II but is also less detailed in some cases. Many of our house officers and students have found it very helpful when faced with the emergency admission of a child with an entity they had not previously encountered. Rapid perusal of the discussion in this section has enabled them to advise referring physicians regarding proper transportation, to direct resuscitative and diagnostic efforts intelligently, and to outline to the parents an overall management plan and prognosis.

This is not intended to be an in-depth discussion of these anomalies. Rather, it is a management outline. Those entities not detailed more extensively in Section II can be studied in texts[1–3] and the literature after the critical initial management has been accomplished. This outline assumes prior assimilation of the important factors in the overall care of the infant from Section I. Factors of singular importance to an individual anomaly are stressed under the headings "Resuscitation and Transportation Requirements" and "Proper Handling." It is assumed that all factors of importance in the general care of the infant such as maintaining body temperature will be applied as well.

DIAPHRAGMATIC HERNIA—BOCHDALEK

This congenital anomaly is a failure of development of the posterior and posterolateral aspects of the diaphragm. It is a defect of the pleuroperitoneal canal fusion and usually results in an open hole without a sac.

USUAL PRESENTATION

1. Respiratory distress includes dyspnea, cyanosis, and shock.
2. Heart sounds are usually heard best in the right chest.

3. The breath sounds are decreased in the left chest.

4. The abdomen is scaphoid and empty.

The above findings assume that the defect is in the left diaphragm. This is the usual case, only one in ten hernias occurring on the right side.[4]

The severity of symptoms and the age of onset depend on the degree of interference with ventilation, particularly of the contralateral lung. Equally important is the interference with venous return to the heart, and consequently with cardiac output, caused by compression and shifting of the mediastinum.

When ventilatory and circulatory capacities are markedly compromised, the baby presents with severe collapse within minutes to hours of birth. The initial Apgar is low and fails to improve. These children face a mortality of 80 to 90 percent if the condition is not corrected immediately. When ventilatory and circulatory interference are minimal, the infant may show no symptoms for days or months, and the anomaly may be diagnosed incidental to evaluation for other respiratory problems such as bronchitis.

DIAGNOSTIC TESTS

A plain, preferably portable, chest x-ray is usually diagnostic. The abdomen should be included on the film. Loops of bowel are seen in the chest; the mediastinum is shifted toward the contralateral side; and no diaphragm is discernible (Fig. 34). If a normal bowel gas pattern is present in the abdomen, the diagnosis should be questioned.

Differential diagnosis includes (a) eventration of a hemidiaphragm, (b) congenital cystic adenomatoid degeneration of the lung, (c) lobar emphysema, (d) staphylococcal pneumonia with pneumatoceles, or (e) other diaphragmatic defects, namely, paraesophageal (hiatal) defects and foramen of Morgagni.

Fortunately, none of these usually causes severe collapse in the first few hours of life, so that it is reasonably safe to assume that an entity associated with severe cardiorespiratory collapse in the immediate few hours after birth that looks like a diaphragmatic hernia will prove to be one. Additional diagnostic maneuvers such as contrast studies of the bowel are contraindicated by the unstable condition of these infants.

When a more stable and usually older infant is found to have a lesion suggestive of diaphragmatic hernia, differentiation from these other entities is essential for proper management and correct choice of surgical procedures. The following points apply:

1. Eventration of a hemidraphragm is associated with less mediastinal shift, less severe ventilatory compromise, and a normal bowel gas pattern, except for a high gastric bubble and splenic flexure of the colon (Fig. 35). A

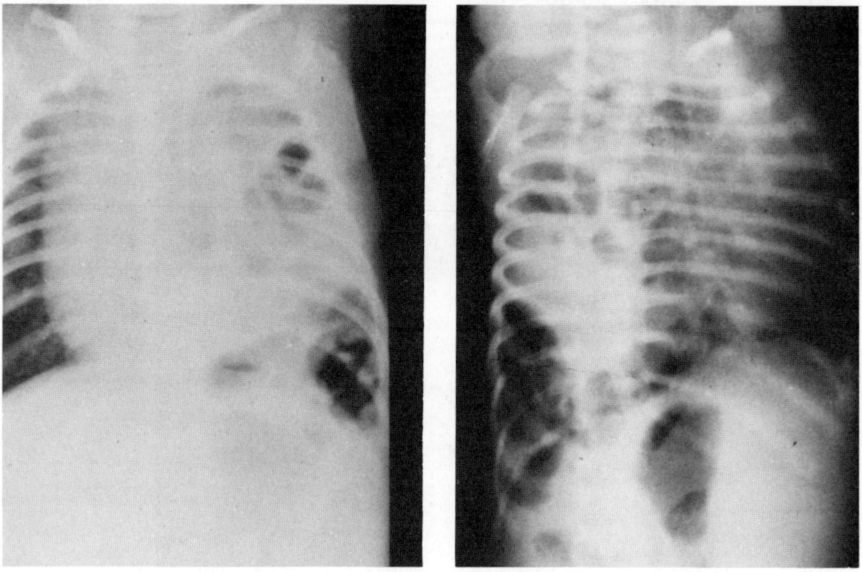

FIG. 34. Anteroposterior and lateral radiographs of infant with left diaphragmatic hernia (Bochdalek) showing bowel gas pattern in left chest, mediastinal shift, and sparse abdominal bowel gas.

plain lateral x-ray will usually define the configurations of the two hemidiaphragms (Fig. 36), and an upper gastrointestinal contrast study will confirm the subdiaphragmatic position of the stomach.

2. Congenital adenomatoid degeneration of the lungs usually involves other lobes of the lung. Early cardiorespiratory collapse is unusual. Symptoms have a more insidious onset. Upper gastrointestinal studies should be done if there is doubt concerning the diagnosis. The bowel gas pattern in the abdomen is normal.

3. Lobar emphysema of the left lower lobe can look like a gastric air shadow above the diaphragm. Plain anteroposterior and lateral x-rays with a radiopaque tube in the stomach will define the diaphragm and confirm that the stomach is properly positioned beneath it.

4. Pneumatoceles in the left lower lobe may occasionally cause staphylococcal pneumonia to be confused with diaphragmatic hernia (Fig. 37). The absence of mediastinal shift, the presence of a normal abdominal gas pattern, the usual symptoms of pneumonia, and the late onset of the problem help to define it. This is not a problem of the immediate newborn period. The baby is stable and if necessary can tolerate contrast gastrointestinal studies to avoid diagnostic and therapeutic errors.

5. Diaphragmatic herniations through the hiatus of the anterior midline

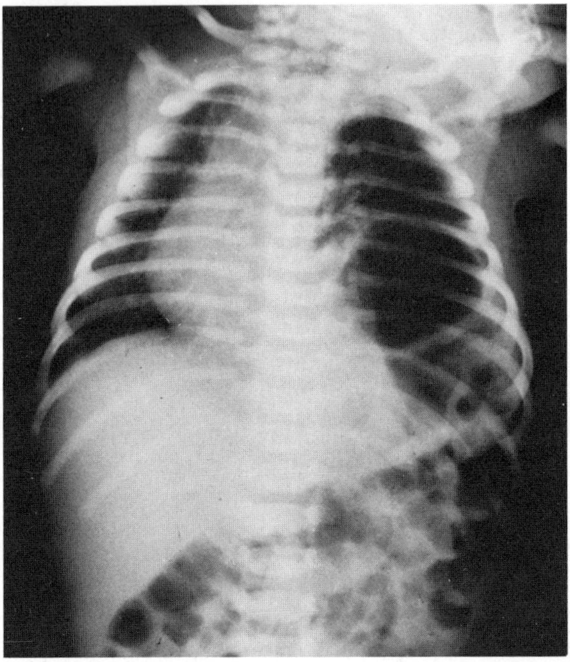

FIG. 35. Radiograph of infant with eventration of left hemidiaphragm showing high gastric bubble, some mediastinal shift, and normal abdominal gas pattern.

foramina of Morgagni are rare in the infant and do not produce symptoms of cardiorespiratory collapse.[4] Hiatal hernias, when associated with reflux of gastric contents, present with vomiting and aspiration pneumonia. Acute aspiration may lead to asphyxial episodes with cyanosis, the so-called dying spells. Volvulus of the stomach has occurred when this organ has herniated through the paraesophageal hiatus.

RESUSCITATION AND TRANSPORTATION REQUIREMENTS

The infant who is in trouble immediately will probably not survive unless expert resuscitation is provided. Cardiorespiratory collapse must be prevented, or else irreversible cellular injury will result. As soon as the diagnosis is suspected, a nasogastric tube must be passed and the gastrointestinal tract kept decompressed to prevent further distention of bowel from increasing the ventilatory and circulatory compromise. Ventilatory support must be provided as needed but must be carefully individualized.

Ventilation by bag and mask is generally contraindicated because it will force air into the stomach. Admittedly, it is better than no ventilation at all, but it may produce irreparable overexpansion of the gastrointestinal tract. Unfortunately, this lesion is so lethal when severe compromise of ventilation and circulation is allowed to occur, that there is no room for any errors or temporizing procedures in resuscitating these infants.

If the baby can ventilate without assistance, oxygen should be provided and preparations made for endotracheal intubation. Assisted ventilation by tube has its own hazards with this lesion. The lungs, especially the hypoplastic ipsilateral lung, are fragile and easily ruptured during assisted ventilation. Some advise prophylactic tube thoracostomies *bilaterally* to avoid superimposing tension pneumothorax on the infant's already compromised ventilation.

Equipment for emergency tube thoracostomies should be at hand, and decompression should be accomplished immediately if the infant deteriorates suddenly after stabilized assisted ventilation has been established.

An intravenous cannula should be inserted, and the baby's circulatory state maintained to provide satisfactory perfusion of vital organs. There are no un-

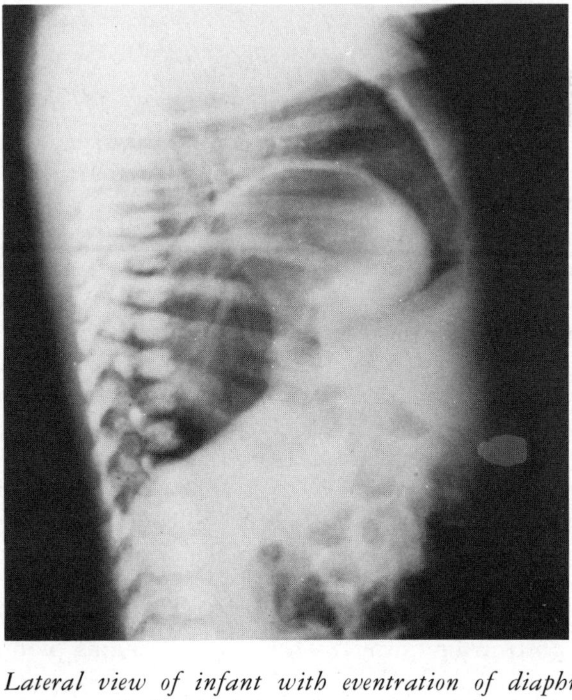

FIG. 36. Lateral view of infant with eventration of diaphragm. Involved hemidiaphragm is seen "ballooning" into chest with gastric air shadow beneath it. Again note abundant abdominal gas pattern.

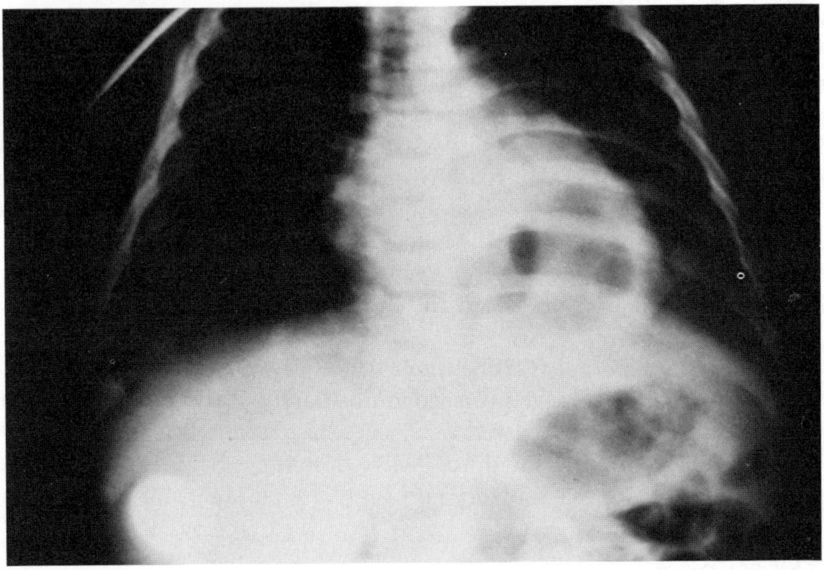

FIG. 37. Pneumatoceles in left lower lobe may be confused with diaphragmatic hernia. Note absence of mediastinal shift. Further evaluation with contrast studies of the intestinal tract if necessary will confirm the diagnosis.

usual losses to account for in these infants unless they have sustained severe ischemic tissue injury. Then the loss of capillary integrity will lead to marked sequestration of fluid in the interstitial spaces with further circulatory collapse and ischemia.

Ideally, the efficiency of the baby's oxygenation and ventilation should be directly monitored by arterial cannulation and frequent sampling of blood gases. Adjustments in assisted ventilation and vascular volume support can then be based on this solid information. Bicarbonate should be administered as needed in response to sustained metabolic acidosis, but this will not correct the acidosis of an uncorrected ventilatory insufficiency.

If the above resuscitative efforts can be successfully accomplished, a stable baby can now be transported for definitive surgical care. Positioning to avoid compression of the side opposite the hernia and continued decompression of the stomach by a well-functioning tube are mandatory during transport.

Unfortunately, the skills, knowledge, and good judgment required to achieve the resuscitative program outlined above are generally not available in the average postpartum nursery. These are challenging problems even for the most experienced neonatologists and pediatric surgeons. Attempts by an inexperienced pediatrician to perform such an extensive resuscitative program usually lead to mistakes, delay, and consequent further ischemic injury. On the other hand, transportation of an unstable infant results in ongoing ischemic injury during transportation.

It should be obvious from the above why the mortality rate is so high for infants symptomatic in the early hours of life. The neonatal center usually receives an infant who has sustained such severe embarrassment of ventilation and perfusion that cellular ischemia has been present for an inordinate length of time. Heroic resuscitative efforts and surgical correction at this point are usually too late, and early death results.

The mechanisms of the postoperative pathophysiology commonly seen with this anomaly are detailed in Section 2 and should be reviewed.

Obviously, some compromise that will offer survival to some of these infants is essential. Honest self-evaluation by the referring physician is essential to determine how far he is capable of pursuing a resuscitative program. Minimum resuscitation should include the following:

1. Effective gastric decompression by a large, well-functioning tube, the continuous function of which must be ensured during transport.
2. Provision of increased environmental oxygen by mask or hood, but without mask and bag ventilatory assistance.
3. Attended transport with proper positioning and provisions for emergency intubation and assisted ventilation as needed.

These maneuvers, when combined with early diagnosis and rapid transport, will allow those babies to survive who can sustain themselves without overly severe ischemic injury for a short period of time. They will be insufficient for the infant whose ventilatory and circulatory functions are severely compromised immediately after birth. They will avoid delay and decompensation of the baby who becomes compromised more gradually. Presently, many of these better infants deteriorate while awaiting transportation or during inept and unsuccessful resuscitative efforts. Unfortunately, a large percentage of infants with diaphragmatic hernias will continue to die if they are not attended to immediately by an experienced neonatal physician.

PROPER HANDLING

All of the factors important for initial resuscitation and transportation also apply to the preoperative handling of these infants. Whatever has not been accomplished in resuscitating and stabilizing the baby should be completed. Ventilatory and circulatory sufficiency should be achieved and acidosis corrected prior to surgery if possible, but occasionally progress is limited until the lung compression and mediastinal shift are surgically alleviated.

CHOICE OF SURGICAL PROCEDURES

Proponents of the transthoracic and transabdominal approaches tend to be adamant in their preferences. Each has its particular advantages, and either can be successful in experienced hands.

The transthoracic route[5] allows the most rapid and immediate decompression of the chest with correction of the obstructed ventilatory and circulatory systems. A sac of peritoneum is easily recognized. These are only occasionally present. Exposure is excellent, but recognition of the posterior diaphragmatic remnant is sometimes difficult. If there is insufficient room in the abdomen to contain the viscera, a secondary abdominal incision will be required for construction of a prosthetic pouch.

The transabdominal approach[6] takes slightly longer, and a peritoneal hernia sac may be missed. However, it provides easy recognition of the margins of the defect. Suturing is facilitated since the bowel can be eviscerated, removing it from the vicinity of the repair. The invariably associated malrotation (actually a total nonfixation) of the intestines can be treated with a Ladd procedure.[7] The importance of this has probably been overstated by proponents of the abdominal approach, however. With either approach, adhesions are probably extensive enough to prevent subsequent volvulus of the malfixed bowel. The most significant advantage of the abdominal approach is that one incision will allow repair of the hernia and also allow construction of a pouch for the viscera if closure produces ventilatory embarrassment from overly high intra-abdominal pressure.

FACTORS OF IMPORTANCE IN POSTOPERATIVE CARE

If a chest tube is used, it should be placed to balanced underwater drainage without suction.[8] No attempts should be made to expand the hypoplastic ipsilateral lung forcefully by either direct ventilation or suction decompression of the pleural space. The lung will expand gradually on its own, and the mediastinum will shift back toward a midline position.

Adequate fluid must be replaced to maintain vascular volume at levels commensurate with good tissue perfusion, but overload should be carefully avoided. All the considerations about intravascular oncotic pressure maintenance with compensation for losses through capillary walls damaged by ischemia apply to these babies.

Assisted ventilation, increased inspired oxygen levels, and positive airway pressure (PEEP or CPAP) are often required. The risk of pneumothorax and need for tube thoracostomy discussed above should be remembered.

Monitoring of vital signs, central pressure, and arterial blood gases is essential so that mechanisms for obtaining this information readily must be available.

Pharmacologic support and manipulation of cardiac, renal and vascular volume modalities may be needed. This may include the use of digitalis derivatives, diuretics, and vasoactive substances such as dopamine.

ASSOCIATED ANOMALIES

This is usually an isolated entity unless it is part of an overall picture of multiple, severe congenital anomalies such as some of the major chromosomal aberrations.

PROGNOSIS

For the baby who is born with respiratory impairment and is immediately symptomatic, the chance of survival is poor unless an almost perfect resuscitative effort is accomplished without delay. A few of these babies have such hypoplastic lungs bilaterally as to be unsalvagable. Most die because stability and surgical correction cannot be achieved with sufficient speed.

The baby who presents with symptoms after 24 hours of life and becomes compromised more slowly has an excellent prognosis if the diagnosis is rapidly confirmed and surgical correction achieved before cardiopulmonary decompensation progresses.

DISCUSSION

Most of what is essential in the care of these infants is discussed above or in Section 2. Although this anomaly has a discouragingly high mortality, continued striving toward salvaging these infants is worth the effort because, if properly corrected before severe ischemic damage results, a normal life can be anticipated for them.

ESOPHAGEAL ATRESIA WITH DISTAL TRACHEOESOPHAGEAL FISTULA

This is the most common variety of these anomalies, being found in about 90 percent of cases.[9] The upper esophagus ends in a blind pouch, usually in the superior mediastinum at about the T_3 level. The fistula is between the distal esophagus and the tracheobronchial tree, usually entering the posterior membranous portion of the trachea just above the carina. Thus, the stomach is directly connected to the airway so that gastric juice can reflux into it freely.

USUAL PRESENTATION

A newborn infant presents with increased "mucus" or saliva. Swallowing difficulties develop, and respiratory distress and cyanosis occur with feedings. Abdominal distention may be present. A history of maternal hydramnios is common.

DIAGNOSTIC TESTS

Attempt to pass a radiopaque nasogastric tube into the stomach; note where it stops. Aspirate and note character of aspirate. Inject air and clamp. Obtain a plain x-ray that includes the neck, chest, and abdomen (see Fig. 25).

The tube is usually found to have stopped in the upper mediastinum, and the dilated air-filled esophageal pouch will be seen extending into the mediastinum from the neck. Gas is present in the abdomen, demonstrating the presence of the tracheoesophageal fistula. Careful note of the gas pattern should be made to identify an associated duodenal atresia if present. As time passes, the abdomen becomes hyperaerated and quite distended.

Contrast media should not be injected into the upper pouch. It is an unnecessary and frequently hazardous step, for the material may be regurgitated from the blind esophagus and aspirated into the larynx.[10]

RESUSCITATION AND TRANSPORTATION REQUIREMENTS

Once the diagnosis is suspected, the baby should be maintained prone and in the head-elevated position. This will help to prevent reflux of gastric juice from the stomach to the lungs through the fistula. Once the diagnosis is confirmed, the pouch tube should be maintained on *continuous* suction for decompression and prevention of aspiration of saliva. Transportation should be expedited, and a knowledgeable attendant should accompany the baby. The prone, head-elevated position should be maintained and continuous suction applied to the pouch tube.

PROPER HANDLING

Maintain the prone, head-elevated position as much as possible during the preoperative evaluation. Continue suction to the pouch tube. Intravenous rehydration will be important if the diagnosis has been missed for several days and the baby has been losing saliva and insensible fluid volumes without replacement.

Establish either an indwelling umbilical or radial artery catheter, so that arterial blood gases can be readily obtained. The choice of surgical procedures will be based on these results (see below), so accurate values are essential. Percutaneous needle puncture for obtaining arterial blood samples may give spurious results if the baby is crying or holding his breath during the painful puncture and may lead to the wrong choice of treatment.

Provide increased inspired oxygen and ventilatory assistance if needed. Begin ultrasonic nebulized mist, since all of these babies have some degree of aspiration of gastric contents. Because soilage of the mediastinum will occur when the esophagus is repaired, begin antibiotics.

CHOICE OF SURGICAL PROCEDURES

1. Urgent: Decompression of gastrointestinal tract.
2. Alternatives:
   a. Gastrostomy under local anesthesia.
   b. Primary repair: Transthoracic extrapleural division and suture of fistula with end-to-end esophagoesophagostomy.
   c. Optional primary repair: Transthoracic extrapleural ligation of fistula and end-to-side in-continuity anastomosis of esophageal segments.[11,12] This procedure has been associated with a high incidence of recurrent fistulas.[13]
   d. Factors in decision: A gastrostomy should be elected unless the following criteria are satisfied:
      (1) The chest is clear to auscultation and x-ray.
      (2) The arterial Po_2 is 60 mm Hg or better in room air.
      (3) Adequate operative, anesthetic, and postoperative pulmonary support are readily available.

      Note that size and prematurity are no longer major determinants.[14]

FACTORS OF IMPORTANCE IN POSTOPERATIVE CARE

1. Keep the neck flexed. Do not hyperextend.
2. Maintain a high level of mist by ultrasonic nebulization. Reduce maintenance fluid amounts appropriately.
3. Daily or twice daily intubation with lavage of the tracheobronchial tree may be needed to clear secretions. The decision to do this requires sound judgment. Ultrasonic mist often obviates the need for this.
4. Maintain an extrapleural tube until a barium swallow confirms an intact open anastomosis at day 5, and oral feedings have been tolerated for 24 hours thereafter.
5. Maintain antibiotic coverage until the chest tube has been removed.
6. Hold gastrostomy or nasogastric tube feedings until the anastomosis is proved to be intact. These infants will invariably reflux from the stomach if fed by tube. If a leak in the anastomosis develops, soilage will occur.
7. If the fifth postoperative day barium swallow is normal, begin oral feedings and remove the stenting nasogastric tube.
8. Continue careful handling and head control to prevent hyperextension of the neck and injury to the anastomosis.
9. Keep the child seated upright continuously to prevent esophageal reflux and aspiration pneumonia.[15]
10. Long-term management requires follow-up for anastomotic stricture.

ASSOCIATED ANOMALIES

Congenital heart anomalies may be present frequently; half of these are serious. Imperforate anus and duodenal atresia occur more frequently than by random association.

PROGNOSIS

Preoperative Condition	Survival (%)
No pneumonia, no cardiac anomalies	90–100
Preoperative pneumonia, unresolved before definitive surgery	50
Pneumonia and prematurity, baby under 1800 g	30–50
Severe congenital heart anomalies	0–25

DISCUSSION

One of the most important factors in better salvage of these infants is proper preoperative handling. Early diagnosis and then proper positioning to prevent gastric reflux to the tracheobronchial tree, combined with suction aspiration of the proximal pouch and avoiding the use of contrast material in making the diagnosis, all help prevent aspiration pneumonia.

If pneumonia is already present as determined either clinically or by x-ray, definitive surgery should be delayed. Gastrostomy should be performed under local anesthesia and intensive pulmonary care instituted combining physiotherapy and ultrasonic nebulization with daily intubations, lavage, and aspiration to clear the lungs. Antibiotic coverage should be instituted. Seven to fourteen days should be allowed to improve the pulmonary status before undertaking definitive repair. More time may be needed, of course, if the pneumonia is slow to clear. The criteria cited above for primary repair, including PO_2 greater than 60 mm Hg in room air must be satisfied.

Tracheostomy may be a very important aid in clearing preoperative pneumonia. The fistula acts as a vent for the pressure that must be generated intratracheally for an effective cough and thus interferes with effective cleaning of secretions. When the pneumonia is slow to clear and secretions are obviously difficult to mobilize, tracheostomy should be performed without hesitation. See Section 1, Chapter 4, for proper management of tracheostomies in infants.

In most babies TPN through central venous catheters will add an important factor of positive nitrogen balance and weight gain. The gastrostomy tube should not be used for feedings while the fistula remains open.

Once such definitive repair is undertaken, a change of antibiotics to include broader gram-negative coverage will better cover the flora at this point. This lesion is also discussed fully in Section 2.

ESOPHAGEAL ATRESIA WITHOUT TRACHEOESOPHAGEAL FISTULA

This is a less common variety, occurring in 5 to 8 percent of all esophageal atresia patients.[9]

USUAL PRESENTATION

A small baby with increased mucus and inability to swallow feedings is born to a mother with hydramnios. The abdomen is flat. Meconium may not be passed normally. Imperforate anus sometimes accompanies this lesion. Cyanosis and dyspnea develop later.

DIAGNOSTIC TESTS

When esophageal atresia is suspected, the exact variety is unknown until after the x-ray is evaluated. Therefore, position the baby head up and prone, so that if a distal tracheoesophageal fistula is present, reflux of gastric juice to the lungs will occur less readily. Pass a large radiopaque nasogastric tube until it stops. Aspirate the tube and note the contents. Inject 50 ml of air and clamp the tube. Obtain a plain x-ray of the baby including the neck, chest, and abdomen. The air-filled pouch containing the tube will be seen in the neck and upper mediastinum. The abdomen will be airless, confirming the absence of a tracheoesophageal fistula (Fig. 38).

RESUSCITATION AND TRANSPORTATION REQUIREMENTS

If this is an isolated anomaly and is diagnosed reasonably early, the baby should remain in good condition. Since gastric contents cannot reflux into the tracheobronchial tree, severe early aspiration pneumonia is less likely to occur. Position considerations are also less important. Maintenance of continuous suction on the pouch tube will prevent aspiration of saliva. General considerations regarding safe transportation of newborn infants apply here.

PROPER HANDLING

Expeditious performance of gastrostomy under local anesthesia will allow early initiation of feedings and avoid complications of a closed-loop obstruction if duodenal atresia is present concomitantly.

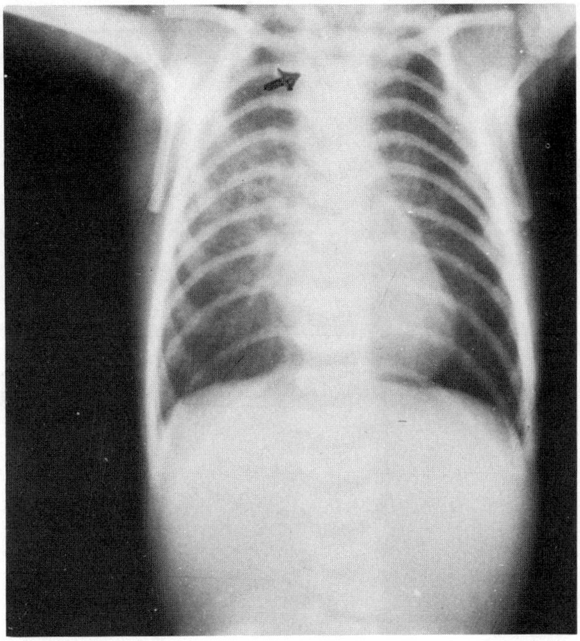

FIG. 38. Babygram of infant with esophageal atresia without tracheoesophageal fistula. Arrow indicates lower limit of blind esophageal pouch. Abdomen is airless. (Courtesy of Dr. Dale Johnson)

CHOICE OF SURGICAL PROCEDURES

The initial procedure for all of these infants should be a gastrostomy. Usually it can be performed under local anesthesia. It may be very difficult, for the "unused" stomach is often quite small.

Barium instilled in the stomach can be made to reflux up the esophagus. Roentgen study will then allow evaluation of the gap between the two esophageal segments. They are rarely close enough for primary anastomosis.

Definitive repair is accomplished by one of four methods:

1. The transverse colon is transposed to the posterior mediastinum through a left thoracotomy (Waterston procedure).[16,17] The left colic vessels from the inferior mesenterics provide the vascular pedicle (Fig. 39). The colon segment is interposed between the two ends of the esophagus, providing a straight conduit and utilizing the cardioesophageal sphincter mechanism to prevent gastroesophageal reflux.

2. The right colon and distal ileum are transposed to the chest in the retrosternal position. The distal end of colon segment is anastomosed to the

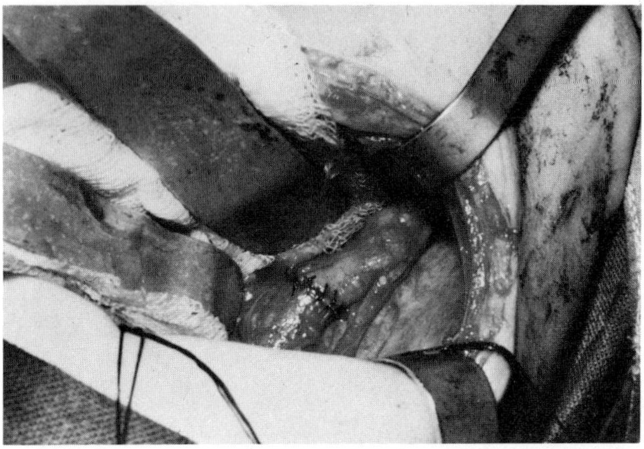

FIG. 39. Operative view of distal coloesophageal anastomosis in Waterston interposition showing vascular pedicle from left colic artery extending into thorax to supply colon segment.

lesser curvature of the stomach, bypassing the cardioesophageal remnant. The advantage of this procedure is the lower morbidity in the event of anastomotic leakage from the extrapleural position of the interposed segment. The roundabout course of the bowel from dorsal esophagus anteriorly to the colon segment and then dorsally again to the stomach makes dilatation and "esophagoscopy" difficult. The smaller diameter of the distal ileum makes the cervical esophagoileal anastomosis easier than the esophagocolonic anastomosis of the Waterston procedure.

3. A gastric tube is formed from the greater curvature of the stomach, transposed to the chest, and anastomosed to the cervical esophagus.[18] The small size of the stomach in these patients may make this difficult. Nevertheless, the procedure, originally devised by Heimlich,[19] has some strong proponents.

4. Recently, Hendren, in cooperation with engineers at the Massachusetts Institute of Technology, has designed an electromagnetic field that can provide intermittent bougienage to the two ends of the esophagus, stretching them toward one another.[20] Metal bougies are placed orally into the cervical esophagus and transgastrically into the distal segment. A transthoracic primary anastomosis can be achieved after about three weeks of this stretching procedure. If this proves to be consistently possible, this should become the procedure of choice since it would avoid interposition procedures that have had significant complications in most people's experience.

If an interposition procedure is elected, cervical esophagostomy should be performed. A right-sided approach is best if a right colon retrosternal procedure is planned. The left side is best for the Waterston procedure and for the Heimlich gastric tube.

FACTORS OF IMPORTANCE IN POSTOPERATIVE CARE

Feedings through the gastrostomy may begin a few days after it is established. Inadvertent dislodging of the tube is a serious hazard to be avoided if possible. If it occurs, great care must be used to ensure that the tube is replaced intragastrically and not intraperitoneally. The latter mistake may be lethal.

Regardless of the type of tube used initially, a smaller Foley catheter is the best choice for replacement. It is passed well into the stomach, the balloon is inflated, and then the balloon is pulled firmly against the stomach wall. This holds the gastric wall against the abdominal wall.

Once the cervical esophagostomy has healed, oral sham feedings should begin. These teach the infant to manipulate and swallow food. They also provide needed oral gratification for the infant.

ASSOCIATED ANOMALIES

Although there is generally a greater coincidence of duodenal atresia and imperforate anus with all types of esophageal atresia, these entities seem to occur more frequently with esophageal atresia without fistula than with the classic variety with associated fistula.

This type of atresia is also more likely to be associated with multiple anomalies and to be seen in association with chromosomal abnormalities such as Trisomy 13/15 or 18. Thus, these severe life-threatening cardiac and renal anomalies more frequently accompany this variant of esophageal atresia.

Finally, malabsorption problems are more common with this type of atresia and may impair normal alimentation after continuity of the gastrointestinal tract is achieved.

PROGNOSIS

Because severe aspiration pneumonia is less common with this variety of esophageal atresia, most infants will survive the newborn period. Long-term survival is reduced however, because of the increased incidence of associated major anomalies in other systems and because the surgical repairs have a higher mortality and morbidity than does the repair of the more common esophageal atresia with fistula.

DISCUSSION

This lesion requires very thoughtful management from its onset. Long-range planning must be started before initial surgical procedures are performed so that the enterotomies can be properly located. Care must be taken during any intra-abdominal procedures not to interfere with the success of subsequent interpositions for reconstruction of the esophagus. Further evaluation of Hendren's imaginative alternative to interposition is essential and may prove to be the optimal approach.

TRACHEOESOPHAGEAL FISTULA WITHOUT ESOPHAGEAL ATRESIA

Only about 1 percent of patients in the general category of esophageal atresia/tracheoesophageal fistula present with this pure fistula variety.[9] The airway and esophagus are intact, but a fistula from the esophagus enters the trachea usually just proximal to the carina.

USUAL PRESENTATION

A newborn infant coughs or gags with feedings, but the esophagus is demonstrated to be patent. Cyanotic spells occur during feedings. Marked abdominal distention is common without any obstructive cause. With diagnostic delay, recurrent aspiration pneumonias are frequent.

DIAGNOSTIC TESTS

Diagnosis by bronchoscopy using the new infant bronchoscope with optical telescopic system* is safe and sure.[21] (Fig. 40). Other approaches, which have been inconsistently successful, include routine bronchoscopy, esophagoscopy, and dye injection studies through tubes positioned in the esophagus at the level of the suspected fistula.[22] Cine-esophagography has been the most successful radiologic procedure in experienced hands. It lacks the direct assurance of modern infant endoscopy, however.

*Karl Storz, Endoscopy-America, Inc., Los Angeles, Calif.

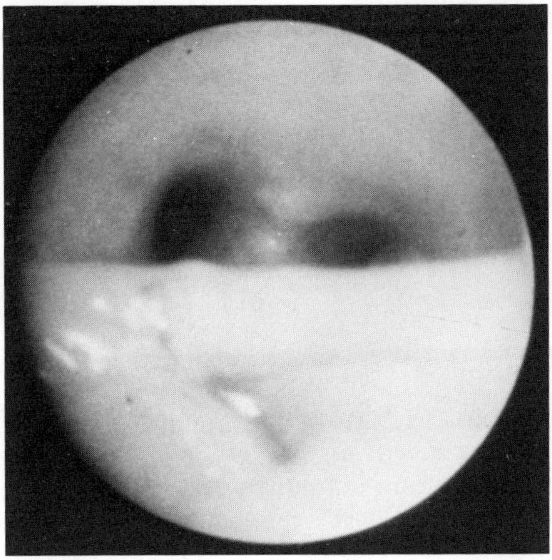

FIG. 40. View of distal trachea and carina through newborn optical telescopic bronchoscope clearly showing a tracheoesophageal fistula in posterior wall of trachea.

RESUSCITATION AND TRANSPORTATION REQUIREMENTS

Unless delay in diagnosis has allowed the development of aspiration pneumonia, no resuscitation is needed except for nasogastric decompression to avoid aspiration. Early transfer of suspect infants for definitive bronchoscopy will prevent morbidity from pneumonia and allow pursuit of other etiologies when no fistula is found in infants with persistent swallowing problems.

PROPER HANDLING

The diagnois should be suspected from the symptoms and pursued thoroughly. The infant should sit up to prevent gastric regurgitation. Small feedings may be tried through the nasogastric tube using the technique of aspiration prior to feeding to avoid overfilling the stomach and resultant esophageal regurgitation.

Aspiration pneumonia, if present, should be treated vigorously employing antibiotics, pulmonary physiotherapy, ultrasonically nebulized mist, and, if necessary, intermittent endotracheal intubation for tracheobronchial lavage and aspiration.

CHOICE OF SURGICAL PROCEDURES

Transcervical division and suture closure of both sides of the fistula are almost always possible.

FACTORS OF IMPORTANCE IN POSTOPERATIVE CARE

Maintain nasogastric tube feedings until an intact closure is demonstrated at six to seven days postoperatively by bronchoscopy and/or barium swallow.

ASSOCIATED ANOMALIES

There are no anomalies usually associated with this entity.

PROGNOSIS

Prognosis is entirely dependent on avoiding severe aspiration pneumonia by early diagnosis. Survival should approach 100 percent. Until recently, mortality from pulmonary decompensation has been very high because diagnostic delay has allowed recurrent pneumonia to ruin the infant's lungs.[22]

DISCUSSION

Careful anesthesia provided by knowledgeable anesthesiologists in infant centers around the country today makes early diagnostic bronchoscopy with telescopic endoscopes the procedure of choice. Any infant presenting with symptoms of dyspnea, gagging, choking, or cyanosis with feedings can be safely referred for evaluation. If this is done, the early diagnosis and correction of this essentially simple lesion should allow achievement of almost 100 percent survival in the future. Other diagnostic methods are no longer warranted, for they are less accurate and only introduce further delay and risk of aspiration.

A brief word about a rare but related anomaly is needed here. Laryngotracheoesophageal cleft may present with symptoms similar to those of tracheoesophageal fistula.[23,24] Early diagnosis is mandatory, both because the soilage is more severe and because the cleft may extend all the way to the main stem bronchi.[25] Again, the modern infant bronchoscope provides the most definitive diagnostic modality.

HYPERTROPHIC PYLORIC STENOSIS

USUAL PRESENTATION

An otherwise healthy baby, usually normal at birth and immediately thereafter, begins to vomit feedings at 2 to 3 weeks of age or slightly later. Onset is rarely beyond the age of 3 months. The vomitus is almost never bile stained. With time, it becomes more projectile in character. Dehydration with attendant decreases in urine and stool output supervenes if diagnosis is delayed. However, until severe hypovolemia is present, these children remain vigorous and accept another feeding immediately after vomiting. They seem to be angry rather than ill. Historically, the first-child and male predominance factors have been overemphasized.

DIAGNOSTIC TESTS

Observe the abdomen for left upper quadrant peristaltic waves. Aspirate the stomach until empty with a nasogastric tube. Note the volume and character of contents in relation to the time after the last feeding. Once the stomach is empty, administer glucose water and palpate for a characteristic "tumor." This must be differentiated from liver edge, colon, pancreas, and kidney.

Upper gastrointestinal x-rays may help to rule out this or other lesions if the "tumor" cannot be felt. False positive results on upper gastrointestinal x-rays are not unusual and may be associated with achalasia or other esophageal dysmotility problems.

RESUSCITATION AND TRANSPORTATION REQUIREMENTS

There are no special requirements.

PROPER HANDLING

These babies are usually moderately dehydrated. Intravenous fluids given overnight prior to surgery are essential for optimal preparation. Unless the baby is severely dehydrated, giving an amount of D_5/½NS + 30 mEq KCl per liter equal to 1.5 times the 24-hour maintenance amount will suffice. This should be given at a rate to infuse this total between admission and surgery. If the baby is more severely dehydrated a longer period of preoperative hydration will be required to administer greater volumes and correct electrolyte abnormalities; D_5/NS with KCl may be required.

These babies frequently seem able to adjust electrolyte concentrations in the face of obvious dehydration and emesis and will be hyposmolar postoperatively if treated with more hypotonic solutions.

When the child is clinically dehydrated, a rapid push of 20 ml/kg of the chosen solution should be given as soon as the intravenous line is in. Nasogastric decompression prevents gastric dilatation and persistent emesis and allows the baby to rest overnight.

CHOICE OF SURGICAL PROCEDURES

The Ramstedt–Friedet–Weber pyloromyotomy is the standard procedure through any of several incisions. An adequate incision onto the gastric surface is important.[26] This is best done by incising only the serosal layer of the pylorus and then "cracking" through the "tumor" to the mucosa with the scalpel handle (Fig. 41). If properly done, no cutting or spreading is necessary and the mucosa is never entered. Avoid entering the bowel lumen. Subcuticular 5/0 chromic is used to close the skin, leaving a cosmetically acceptable scar.

FACTORS OF IMPORTANCE IN POSTOPERATIVE CARE

The nasogastric tube may be removed in the recovery room. Feedings should be started in 6 hours. Small, frequent feedings are gradually increased in volume and changed from D_5/water to formula.

A basic rule to follow is: Do not change quantity and content at the same time. Aim to have the baby on full formula feedings by the third postoperative day if possible. Discharge varies from three to five days postoperatively.

ASSOCIATED ANOMALIES

There are no anomalies commonly associated with this lesion.

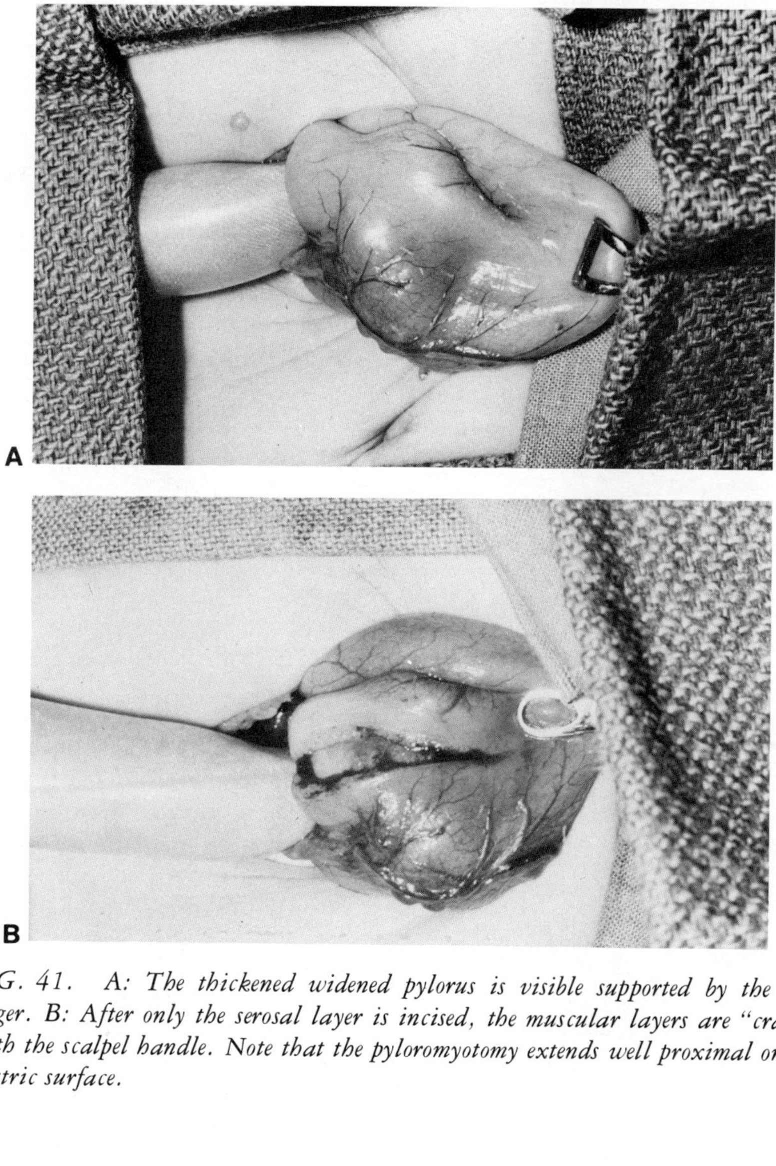

FIG. 41. A: The thickened widened pylorus is visible supported by the index finger. B: After only the serosal layer is incised, the muscular layers are "cracked" with the scalpel handle. Note that the pyloromyotomy extends well proximal onto the gastric surface.

PROGNOSIS

Prognosis is excellent. This is probably the most satisfying and uncomplicated lesion to treat in pediatric surgery.

DISCUSSION

Pyloric stenosis is very rarely seen in the age group under 1 to 2 weeks of age and almost never in the immediate neonatal period. Achalasia or chalasia can produce emesis of primarily gastric contents, and x-rays may show pylorospasm. Insisting on palpating the tumor prior to surgery will prevent embarrassing errors and unnecessary surgery.

If the mucosa is inadvertently entered during pyloromyotomy, the entire pyloric incision should be carefully and fully closed and a piece of omentum should be tacked up to it. The pylorus should then be rotated and a new pylorotomy performed. Closing only the hole in the mucosa will usually lead to perforation, soilage, and peritonitis. When the pyloromyotomy is performed with the "cracking technique" mentioned above this complication rarely occurs.

DUODENAL OBSTRUCTIONS

Duodenal obstructions include malrotation, duodenal atresia, duodenal stenosis, annular pancreas, and intrinsic webs, complete or incomplete. The main consideration is to differentiate between the potentially rapidly lethal entity of malrotation with volvulus and mesenteric strangulation, and the chronic congenital obstructions such as duodenal atresia or annular pancreas.

USUAL PRESENTATION

With complete obstructions, the newborn vomits green and has bile-stained gastric aspirates. Feedings are vomited. Abdominal distention is limited to the left upper quadrant. Meconium may or may not be passed.

With incomplete obstructions, intermittent green emesis is associated with minimal abdominal distention. Usually meconium and gas are passed, and often early feedings are tolerated, but obstruction may supervene when full formula is begun. Months or years may go by without symptoms.

DIAGNOSTIC TESTS

When the symptoms present in the immediate newborn period, pass a nasogastric tube, empty the stomach, inject 40 to 50 ml of air, clamp the tube, and obtain supine, upright, and lateral films of the chest and abdomen. Evaluation of these will determine the need for further studies.

Air is an excellent contrast medium for proximal bowel obstructions. Here the main consideration is to rule out malrotation. This is the most serious life-threatening obstructive entity of childhood, and, unless it is ruled out, evaluation and surgical exploration must be done urgently. If air demonstrates complete duodenal obstruction and the duodenum is dilated, this is the so-called double-bubble film usually indicative of duodenal atresia or a completely obstructing annular pancreas. However, complete duodenal obstruction from malrotation may have been present in utero and present with identical appearances. Emergency surgery is indicated to avoid this mistake. If delay of surgery is desirable because of the unstable condition of the baby, for instance, if respiratory distress complicates the picture, a barium enema may be helpful. If the course of the colon is completely normal, delay until the baby improves is probably safe.

If air demonstrates a partial duodenal obstruction with air beyond the obstruction, malrotation becomes the most likely diagnosis. The next diagnostic maneuver should be an upper gastrointestinal series with barium.[27,28] Only recently has the fact of the upper gastrointestinal nature of malrotation obstruction been emphasized. Classically, a barium enema has been the diagnostic procedure of choice, but this may be inconclusive or confusing.[28] (see Fig. 28).

The findings on an upper gastrointestinal series suggestive of malrotation are an accordionated pattern to the duodenal C loop and failure of the duodenum to cross the spine back to a normal ligament of Treitz, clearly in the left upper quadrant (Fig. 42). On barium enema a right upper quadrant position of the cecum usually with the cecal tip and appendix pointing toward the umbilicus is highly suggestive of malrotation. The true location of the cecum may be very difficult to determine on barium enema, however.

RESUSCITATION AND TRANSPORTATION REQUIREMENTS

Once the diagnosis of upper gastrointestinal obstruction is made, further evaluation is best delayed until the baby reaches the neonatal center. If contrast studies have not already been done, urge early transfer and completion of the diagnostic work-up thereafter.

Unless the baby has aspirated, requiring airway resuscitation and support,

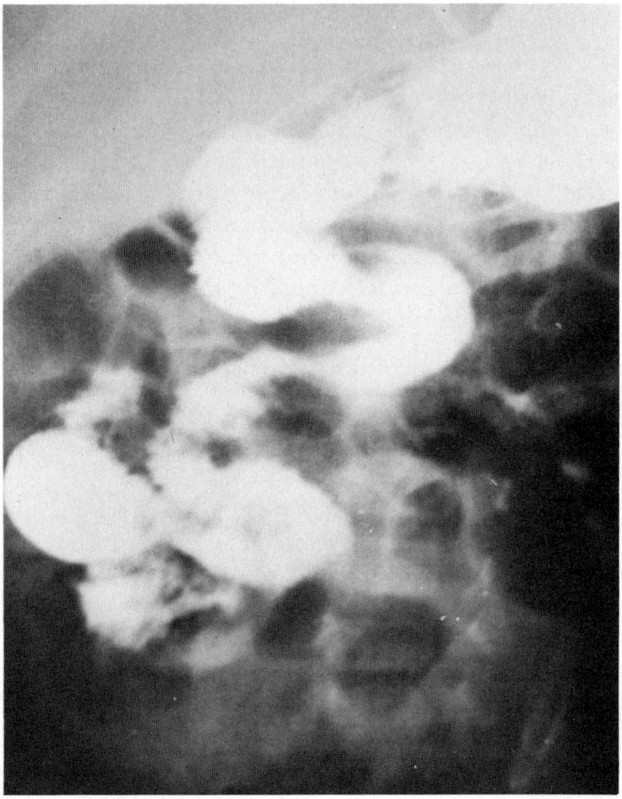

FIG. 42. Upper gastrointestinal radiographic series on infant with malrotation showing abnormal duodenal C loop, failure to cross to left upper quadrant, and jejunum wandering to right of the spine.

nasogastric decompression is the only specific requirement during transport. Delays for initiating intravenous fluid replacement are rarely warranted. Expeditious resuscitation and completion of the diagnostic evaluation can be done best by experienced specialists. Delays may lead to loss of additional bowel if malrotation with strangulating volvulus is the etiology of the obstruction (Fig. 43).

PROPER HANDLING

If after the above diagnostic work-up any doubt as to the diagnosis remains, the patient should be operated on at once, for to miss a strangulating volvulus from malrotation would be a tragedy. (Fig. 44).

For the upper gastrointestinal study, barium should be used. A minimum of dye (4 to 5 ml) should be given by tube. Any excess should be aspirated after the procedure is completed.

Baseline bilirubin studies are advised for all newborn surgical patients, but duodenal and high jejunal atresias are particularly likely to show bilirubin elevations. Often these are more severe postoperatively. This may reflect an interference with enterohepatic circulation or some increased liver malfunction due to low-grade obstruction.

If atresia of the duodenum is diagnosed clearly, a nasogastric tube may be passed and attached to suction and surgery scheduled electively at the first opportunity. Such a delay is warranted only if dictated by the condition of the baby.

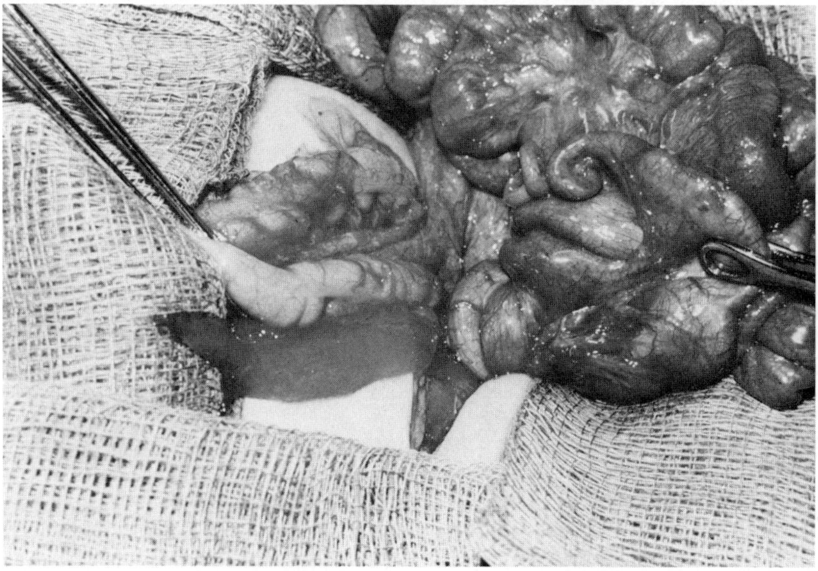

FIG. 43. Operative view of volvulus from malrotation. The transverse colon is held in the forceps at the left. Just to the right of the transverse colon, in the middle of the picture, are the loops of bowel enwrapping the base of the small bowel mesentery. The cecum is held in the forceps at the right, and the appendix can be seen coiling away from it.

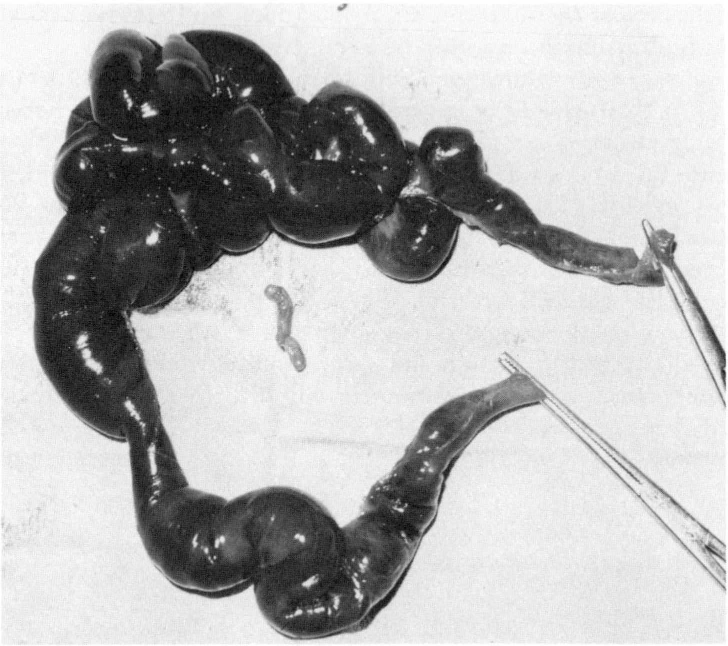

FIG. 44. Large segment of necrotic bowel removed from newborn presenting with obstructed duodenum and found to have malrotation with volvulus and mesenteric strangulation.

CHOICE OF SURGICAL PROCEDURES

1. Duodenal atresia and/or annular pancreas:[29] duodenoplasty, duodenoduodenostomy,[30] or duodenojejunostomy (rarely).
2. Duodenal stenosis or web: duodenoplasty.
3. Malrotation: Ladd procedure:[7] lysis of adhesions, derotation of volvulus, resection of any obviously necrotic bowel. Place the cecum in the left lower quadrant, the duodenum in the right lower quadrant. Incidental appendectomy by the total intussusception technique should be performed[31,32] because the postoperative location of the appendix is uncertain and variable.

FACTORS OF IMPORTANCE IN POSTOPERATIVE CARE

Continue to watch for hyperbilirubinemia and treat appropriately. Albumin, bilirubin lights, and exchange tranfusion may all help.

When drainage from the gastrostomy tube or nasogastric tube decreases significantly, attach a syringe barrel without plunger to the tube. Suspend it above the child and check gastric residuals every 4 hours. Then begin 10 to 15 ml D_5/W or D_5/ ¼NS each hour, aspirating the tube before each feeding and replacing aspirate plus enough feeding to achieve the total desired. These instructions must be given with great care or they may be misinterpreted, resulting usually in discarding the aspirates with resultant electrolyte depletion. Volumes may be advanced stepwise thereafter.

Positioning may be important because of the functionally inefficient, dilated duodenum. Turn the infant to the right side or prone after feedings.

Usually these babies will be functioning well by seven to ten days, but prolonged functional obstruction may occur.

If short bowel or severe ischemia has resulted from strangulating volvulus, a prolonged period of malabsorption may result. Total parenteral nutrition will maintain the baby while small incremental advancements in volume and type of feedings allow gradual healing and adaptation of the remaining bowel.

ASSOCIATED ANOMALIES

1. Malrotation (usually an isolated entity).
2. Duodenal atresia, stenosis, annular pancreas; Down's syndrome in 15 to 30 percent (mongolism).[33,34]
3. Multiple atresias of small bowel rarely occur with duodenal atresia, but patency of the distal gastrointestinal tract should always be demonstrated by instilling saline and mineral oil and flushing it through to the anus.

PROGNOSIS

When these lesions occur as isolated entities, prognosis should be quite good. Malrotation, of course, carries with it the threat of strangulation from mesenteric volvulus, so its prognosis depends on the presence or absence of necrotic intestine.

DISCUSSION

As emphasized above, the most important step in handling a baby with high intestinal obstruction is to rule out malrotation. Generally, malrotation obstructions present with acute onset in the postnatal period and, in this respect, differ from the atresias and annular pancreas. It is very important to grasp the fact that, once a baby has demonstrated complete patency of his gastrointestinal tract by the passage of air or transitional stool through it, the congenital atresias are ruled out forever. Thus, the baby who obstructs after complete air passage has an acute intestinal obstruction, most frequently from an incarcerated inguinal hernia but more seriously from malrotation. Occasionally, but very rarely, such entities as congenital bands, omphalomesenteric ducts, or internal hernias are involved, but the entity that is most life-threatening and that therefore demands early surgery is volvulus from malrotation.

Note that, as discussed below under jejunoileal atresia, the passage of meconium does not rule out congenital atresias; only the passage of air or transitional stool does this. If a clear-cut demonstration of a congenital atresia type of obstruction can be made, surgery need not be urgent, and delays of days or weeks may be allowable, if such will allow improvement of an aspiration pneumonia or respiratory distress syndrome. Total parental nutrition will maintain a positive nitrogen balance and allow reasonable growth and weight gain. Such a delay merely to achieve additional growth and weight gain is not reasonable, however, in view of the risks of infection by central catheters.

SMALL BOWEL ATRESIAS

Small bowel atresias include jejunal atresia, ileal atresia, multiple atresias, and small bowel stenosis. Atresia is by far the more common entity, stenosis being quite rare. The etiology of most, if not all, atresias is an in utero vascular accident.[35] As noted in the discussion, the timing of the accident influences the signs that accompany the lesion. Intussusception of polyps or Meckel's diverticulum may play a causative role. In utero malrotation may be the most common etiology, and persistent volvulus may lead to further loss of intestine in the postnatal period.

USUAL PRESENTATION

A variably distended newborn baby vomits feedings and bile. Loops of dilated bowel are frequently visible and palpable. Rapid dehydration and electrolyte imbalance may occur. Passage of meconium does not rule out these entities.

DIAGNOSTIC TESTS

Passage of a nasogastric tube confirms the nature of the gastric contents and rules out gastric dilatation as the cause of abdominal distention. Abdominal x-rays to include supine, lateral, and upright views show variable numbers of loops of dilated bowel with air fluid levels on the upright film. All loops are dilated to about the same degree. Be aware that one cannot differentiate small from large bowel in infants except when the usual course of the the colon is completely outlined by air, including gas in the pelvic colon. The appearance and pattern of isolated loops will not distinguish small from large bowel in the infant under the age of 2 years. Indeed, even on barium enema the caliber change from cecum to ileum may not be clearly determinable.

RESUSCITATION AND TRANSPORTATION REQUIREMENTS

Adequate nasogastric decompression is essential to prevent aspiration. Further support needs are based on the general condition of the infant.

PROPER HANDLING

Once the diagnosis is suspected, nasogastric decompression must be instituted at once to prevent aspiration pneumonia. The diagnosis can be readily made from plain abdominal films (Fig. 45). No contrast studies are usually needed, especially if urgent surgery is planned. Occasionally, small bowel atresias result from in utero malrotations with strangulating volvulus. Further strangulation may occur in the postnatal period so that, if delay of sugery is being considered, an upper gastrointestinal study should be obtained to be certain that the duodenal C loop and ligament of Treitz are normally located. If doubt exists, surgery probably should not be delayed. We have seen patients for whom such a delay would have resulted in massive additional bowel loss (Fig 46).

Again, attention to bilirubin levels pre- and postoperatively is essential, especially in the more proximal obstructions where low-grade biliary obstruction and interference with the enterohepatic circulation of bile may result in dramatic changes in bilirubin levels. Timing of surgery depends on the condition of the baby. If aspiration pneumonia, respiratory distress syndrome, or sepsis is already present, delay is warranted for thorough treatment as long as malrotation has been ruled out. Adequate gastrointestinal decompression is mandatory during this time to prevent aspiration and overdistention of the bowel loops with necrosis or perforation. If a nasogastric tube is

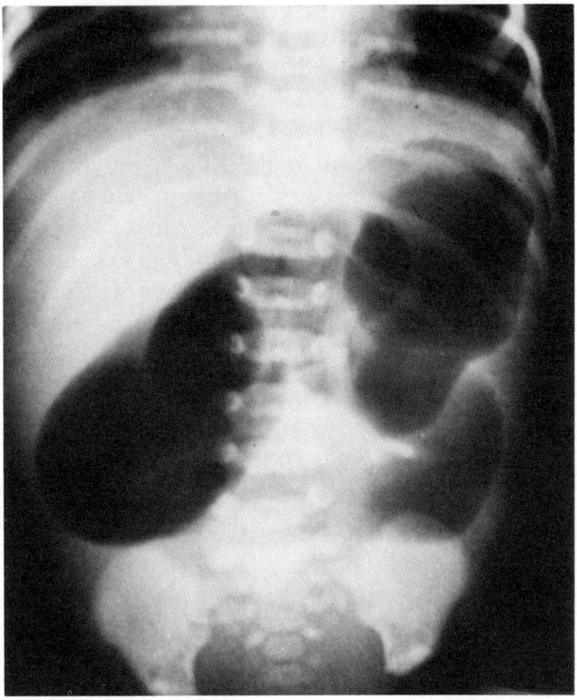

FIG. 45. A typical radiograph of an infant with jejunal atresia showing several loops of dilated, air-filled proximal bowel without distal bowel gas.

insufficient for this purpose, a gastrostomy can be easily performed under local anesthesia. Total parenteral nutritional support during the period of pretreatment is important.

CHOICE OF SURGICAL PROCEDURES

For the usual atresia, resection of the very dilated and functionally inefficient terminal blind-ended loop of the proximal segment contributes significantly to the speed of postoperative functional recovery.[36] An end-to-end one- or two-layer anastomosis is then performed. There will invariably be disparity between the two anastomotic ends. Beveling the distal end obliquely with the antimesenteric side shorter will aid in the performance of the anastomosis, but the functional lumen size will always be limited by the diameter of the distal bowel.

Interrupting all sutures will ensure a more distensible anastomosis and allow for growth. When the atresia is very near the ligament of Treitz such that the duodenum participates in the marked dilation of the terminal blind-ended proximal segment, resection is hazardous, and end-to-end anastomosis between the very dilated proximal segment and the narrow distal segment must be achieved. Here it is essential to place the anastomosis at the very tip of the blind-ended proximal pouch to prevent ballooning of the proximal bowel beyond the anastomosis resulting in a functional obstruction.

It is mandatory that continuity and patency of the lumen of the entire bowel then be demonstrated. This can be readily achieved by the instillation of mineral oil and saline into the distal bowel through a catheter prior to

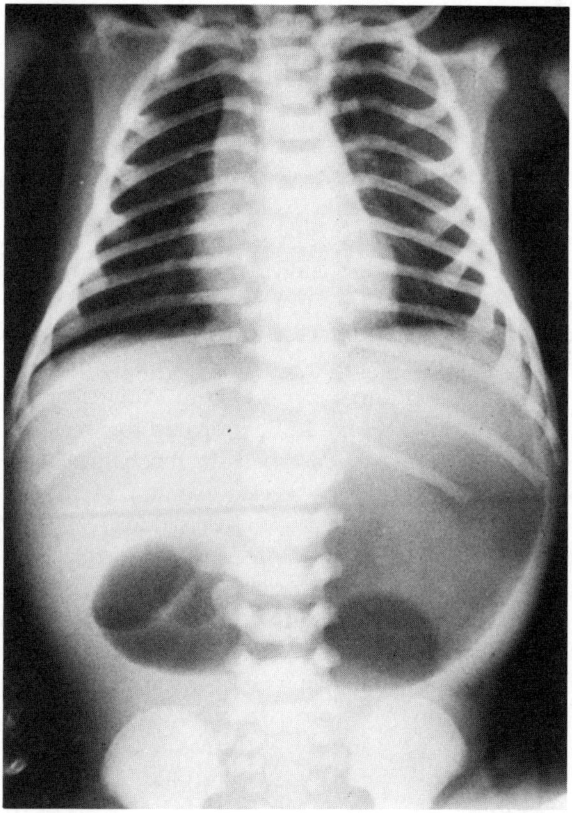

FIG. 46. Radiograph of infant with apparent high jejunal obstruction. At operation an extensive area of atresia due to malrotation with in utero volvulus and strangulation was found. Additional small bowel was acutely compromised and was saved by early surgical intervention.

completion of the anastomosis. The circulating nurse can confirm evacuation of the oil from the baby's anus. This step also serves to avoid postoperative meconium impaction. Appendectomy should be performed.

FACTORS OF IMPORTANCE IN POSTOPERATIVE CARE

As in duodenal atresia, concern for hyperbilirubinemia is essential in the postoperative period. Depending somewhat on whether a large distended segment remains, the period before the bowel begins to function adequately may be quite prolonged. If TPN was begun preoperatively, it should be continued until a full diet is tolerated by the gastrointestinal route. If parenteral alimentation was not begun preoperatively, but there was a delay between birth and surgery of over 48 to 72 hours, parenteral alimentation should be instituted shortly after surgery. If the baby was operated on shortly after birth, a delay of no more than seven to eight days may be tolerated prior to instituting parenteral alimentation, if an adequate peripheral venous line, preferably a plastic cannula,[37] will allow administration of at least 10 percent dextrose solutions and daily albumin. If the gastrointestinal tract is not functioning well by seven to eight days, TPN should be instituted at once. A safe way to begin feedings is with the hanging syringe and aspiration technique described under duodenal atresia.

It is essential to consider all the factors discussed in the general sections on postoperative maintenance and TPN. Include adequate mineral and vitamin supplements, especially sodium and potassium, biweekly plasma supplements, and daily albumin. One should be prepared for weeks and sometimes months of bowel hypofunction even when no mechanical obstruction persists. However, sometime after two weeks, patency of the gastrointestinal tract should be demonstrated by contrast x-ray studies.

A distressing sequel to many of these atresias is the short bowel syndrome.[38] This is an obvious accompaniment of extensive resections, whether for multiple atresias or volvulus with gangrene. When gastrointestinal alimentation is established, the baby develops profuse watery diarrhea and fails to gain weight. Rapid dehydration is a constant threat.

Some babies with seemingly adequate residual bowel length present a similar postoperative picture. Only recently has it been realized that this is often due to a disaccharidase deficiency syndrome similar to the primary malabsorption syndrome of that type.[39] Treatment for all of these problems includes carefully considered formula changes tending toward more simple components such as monosaccharide sugars, amino acid hydrolysates, and medium-chain triglycerides.

ASSOCIATED ANOMALIES

No anomalies are consistently associated with this entity.

PROGNOSIS

If adequate bowel length remains and a satisfactory anastomosis is performed, the chance of survival should be excellent. When short bowel syndrome or other malabsorption problems complicate the postoperative period, survival and adaptation can usually be achieved if the baby can be maintained on TPN for the required time period. Sepsis remains a significant threat to these babies throughout this period of artificial feeding.

MECONIUM ILEUS, MUCOVISCIDOSIS, AND CYSTIC FIBROSIS

This diagnosis means that the baby has cystic fibrosis.[40]

USUAL PRESENTATION

A newborn infant is distended at birth and becomes increasingly so early in the neonatal period. Bile is vomited, and feedings are returned. No meconium is passed, and only mucous plugs are found in the rectum.

A history of cystic fibrosis in the family may or may not be obtainable. Respiratory symptoms or chest x-ray findings of mucoviscidosis are rarely present preoperatively.

DIAGNOSTIC TESTS

Plain films of the abdomen show evidence of a distal bowel obstruction. Unlike the uniform dilatation of the loops found in the simple atresias, there is disparity in the size of the loops, a soap bubble appearance in the lumen representing a mixture of air and meconium, and a sparsity of air–fluid levels on the erect film. This triad of findings is highly suggestive of this lesion[41] (Fig. 47).

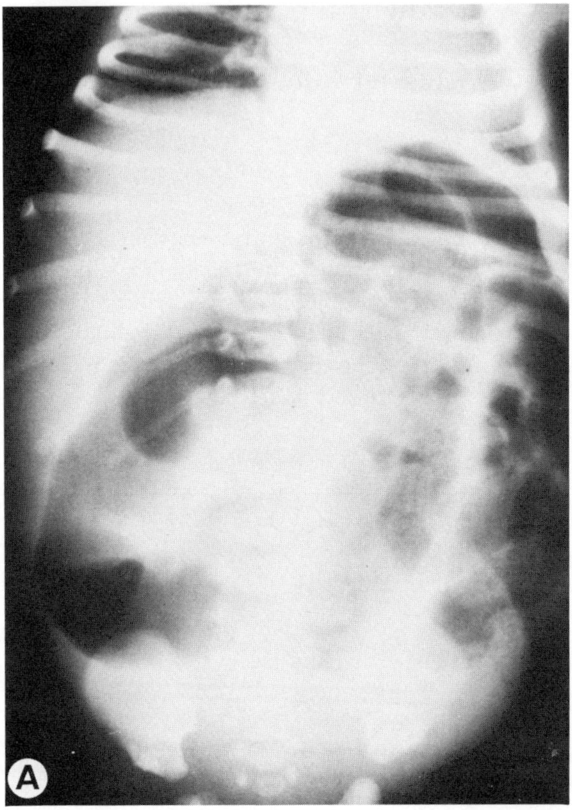

FIG. 47. Plain supine (A) and upright (B) films of the abdomen of a patient with meconium ileus illustrating the triad of findings suggestive of this diagnosis: disparity in the size of the loops, sparsity of air—fluid levels on the upright film, and bubbly appearance of the intraluminal contents.

A water-soluble contrast enema usually shows a "microcolon" with beads of inspissated mucus (Fig. 48). Obstruction is encountered in the distal ileum, and, after two to three fillings and emptying of the enema, the dye refluxes proximal to the obstructed level. Numerous loops of small intestine are filled, and, when this volume is allowed to empty, the inspissated meconium is evacuated.

Sweat chlorides confirm the diagnosis of mucoviscidosis if the level is above 60 mEq/liter. They may be inaccurate in the immediate newborn period, although, generally, positive results are meaningful.

Stool trypsin levels are decreased.

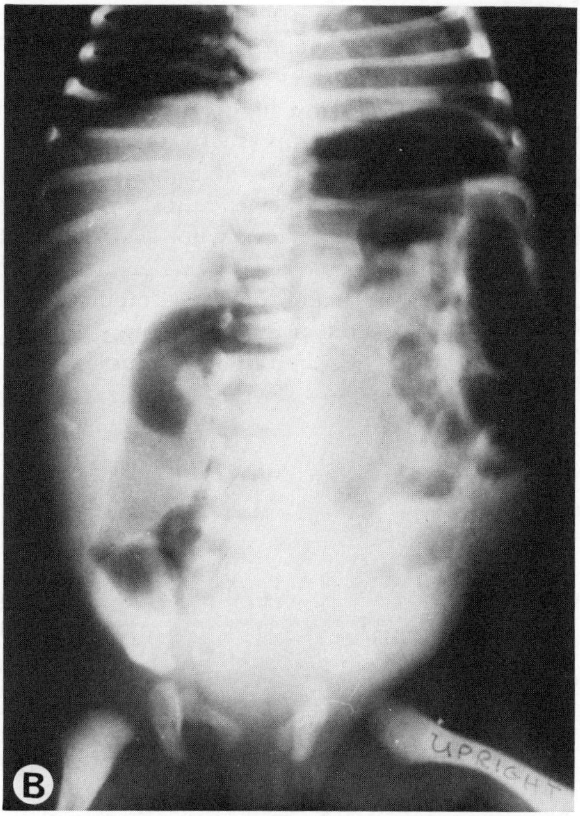

FIG. 47B.

RESUSCITATION AND TRANSPORTATION REQUIREMENTS

The infant should be protected from vomiting and aspirating by tube decompression of the stomach.

PROPER HANDLING

Once the diagnosis is suspected, the baby should be placed in ultrasonic mist, and respiratory physical therapy should be instituted. Broad-spectrum antibiotic coverage is probably warranted.

Repeated administration of water-soluble enemas to relieve the obstruction is safe so long as the baby is given time to rest, recuperate, and achieve fluid and electrolyte correction between times.[42,43]

Water-soluble contrast media have high osmolarities, generally ranging between 1500 and 2000 mOsm compared to 289 mOsm of extracellular fluid. They work by drawing extracellular fluid intraluminally along this osmolar concentration gradient.[44] A dependable intravenous catheter must be in place prior to using water-soluble agents, for a loss of extracellular fluid and vascular volume can be expected due to this great intraluminal shift of fluid. Immediately after instillation of the water-soluble agent, 20 ml/kg of D_5/RL should be given, preferably with 5 percent albumin (5g/100 ml). Then adequate D_5/RL with or without albumin must be administered over

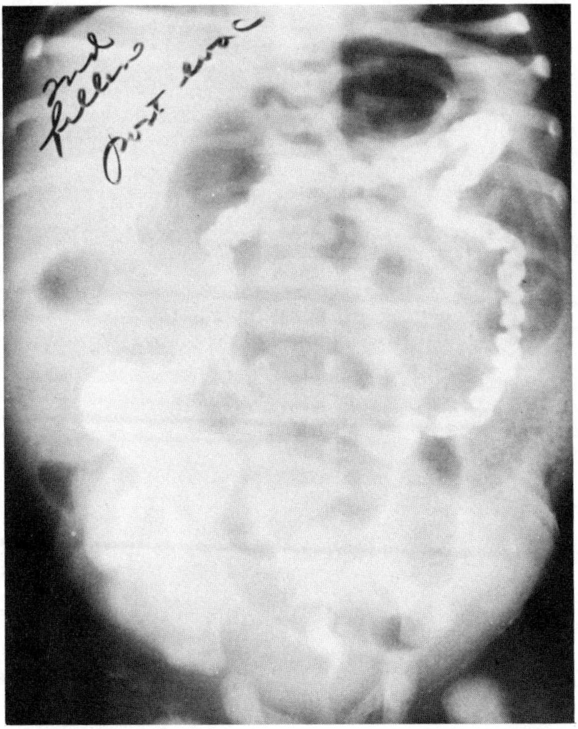

FIG. 48. Water-soluble contrast enema of a patient with meconium ileus showing the unused colon with beaded appearance of inspissated mucus superimposed on the dilated small bowel loops. Repeated fillings and emptying may be needed to reflux the dye into the proximal dilated bowel and achieve emptying of the meconium.

the next 24 hours to maintain adequate urine output of 40 ml/kg per 24 hours, or about 1 to 2 ml/kg per hour. Maintenance fluid must also be given during this period. The most widely used agent, meglumine diatrizoate plus sodium diatrizoate,* is said to contain a small amount of Tween 80,[42,43] a wetting agent that breaks up the adhesion of the meconium to the bowel wall. It should be used full strength and preferably inserted through a balloonless catheter, well-taped in place and pushed in with a large syringe rather than by hydrostatic pressure. Fluoroscopic monitoring is mandatory. Recent reports have questioned the safety of Tween 80 and have suggested the use of water-soluble agents not containing this detergent.[45,46]

The enema treatment is contraindicated by free perforation, atresia, volvulus, and intussusception with failed reduction. It should be abandoned if any of these develop subsequent to its use.

The end point of enema treatment for meconium ileus is reached when reflux well into the dilated small bowel is achieved, adequate meconium is passed and continues to be passed, and relief of the obstruction is demonstrated by follow-up x-rays and continued passage of stool and gas.

Repeated enema treatment is indicated as long as additional meconium is passed and no mechanical obstruction is demonstrated. If complete resolution cannot be achieved, surgery is then required.

CHOICE OF SURGICAL PROCEDURES

When no complicating factor other than failure of enema treatment is present, the goal of surgery is to relieve the inspissation of the meconium with minimal trauma to the bowel. Water-soluble contrast media can sometimes be instilled through a rectal tube while the bowel is exposed and gently milked proximally until it reaches the level of obstruction. If a perforation is present or an enterotomy required, water-soluble media instilled through the enterotomy will loosen the inspissated meconium.

When resection is required or simple enterotomy with irrigation is inadequate, the Bishop–Koop distal ileostomy with end-to-side enteroenterostomy[47] allows resection and primary anastomosis while providing a vent for postoperative washouts with contrast media or *N*-acetylcysteine.[48]

Attempts to "milk" the inspissated meconium along the bowel have usually produced injury to the wall and mesentery. Such an approach should be avoided, as should multiple enterotomies for meconium evacuation.

When perforation, strangulating volvulus, or complete mechanical obstruction are the indications for surgery, these entities must be treated appropriately.

*Gastrografin, Squibb & Sons, E.R., Princeton, N.J.

FACTORS OF IMPORTANCE IN POSTOPERATIVE CARE

1. Continued and persistent washouts of meconium until complete relief of the obstruction is achieved.
2. Vigorous respiratory care including ultrasonic mist, postural drainage, and chest clapping.
3. Antibiotic coverage and frequent cultures of respiratory secretions with appropriate antibiotic changes.
4. Proper management of postoperative diet, initially using a "pre-digested" formula since it requires no pancreatic enzymes for digestion and then adding pancreatic enzymes when more common formulas are used. Lifetime maintenance of pancreatic enzymes is usually required.[49,50] This management program is indicated for either postsurgical or postenema patients.
5. Long-term care of the respiratory component of mucoviscidosis.[50]

ASSOCIATED ANOMALIES

Outside of other systems involved in mucoviscidosis there are no associated anomalies. The former include (a) prolonged and repeated respiratory illnesses, (b) continued deficiencies of digestive enzymes and abnormal gastrointestinal mucus, (c) occasional liver degeneration secondary to enzymatic abnormalities,[51] (d) rectal prolapse, and (e) gastrointestinal bleeding and hypersplenism secondary to liver cirrhosis and portal hypertension.[52]

PROGNOSIS

Prognosis is guarded and is most dependent on long- and short-term respiratory care and management.

INTUSSUSCEPTION

USUAL PRESENTATION

A healthy, well-fed baby between 3 months and 24 months of age has a sudden onset of colicky abdominal pain. The infant frequently draws the legs up in pain, then relaxes completely between colicky episodes. As time passes, signs of gastrointestinal obstruction, vomiting, and abdominal distention appear. The well-known "currant jelly" bloody stools are present in only about 30 percent of cases. Occasionally, intussusception presents in the newborn period,[53] and it is a known cause of atresia in utero.

DIAGNOSTIC TESTS

This is another entity that must be thought of to be diagnosed. A child presenting with this symptom complex deserves early barium enema evaluation. This will make the diagnosis and will frequently be therapeutic.[54]

RESUSCITATION AND TRANSPORTATION REQUIREMENTS

There are no special requirements except to treat severe dehydration and vascular collapse if present.

PROPER HANDLING

Admit the child to the hospital. Establish a well-functioning intravenous line. Resuscitate the infant from dehydration if necessary prior to barium enema. Pass a nasogastric tube and empty the stomach to prevent aspiration pneumonia. The barium enema should be done with the bag at a maximum of 30 to 36 inches above the table. Barium should run freely with minimal manipulation of the bowel. No attempt to force reduction is allowable (Fig. 49). The end point is free reflux into the ileum, demonstrating complete reduction. Several attempts may be made, emptying the bowel between refillings.

If reduction is successful, recheck the abdominal plain film, after emptying the colon, to insure against reintussusception. Observe in hospital until feedings are tolerated, stool is passed, and the infant is asymptomatic. If reduction fails, proceed at once to surgery.

CHOICE OF SURGICAL PROCEDURES

Transabdominal reduction by squeezing the intussusceptum backward (like squeezing toothpaste in a tube) (Fig. 50) is the procedure of choice.[54] The bowel should never be pulled apart. If complete reduction is impossible, resect as necessary. Search for a "lead point" such as a Meckel's diverticulum or polyp, and treat this appropriately. Resect any necrotic bowel and anastomose primarily. Incidental appendectomy is indicated. Occasionally

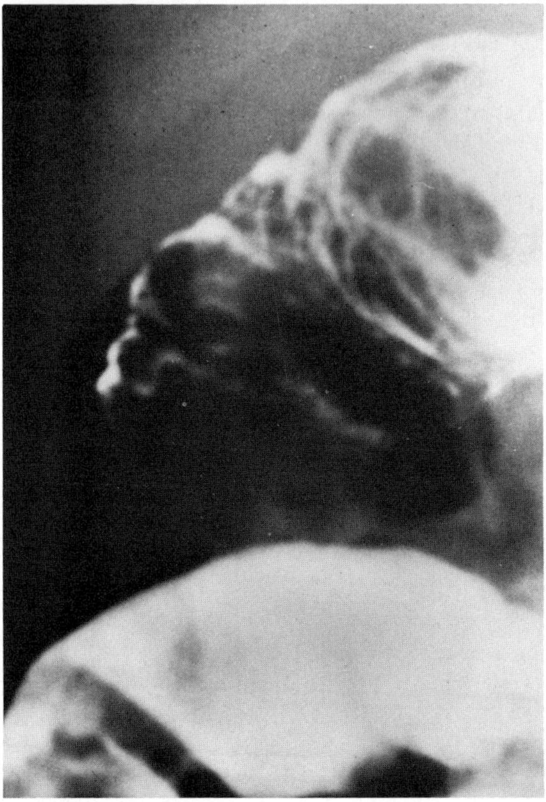

FIG. 49. Coned-down view of hepatic flexure of colon during hydrostatic barium reduction of an intussusception. The intussusceptum is seen within the lumen of the hepatic flexure outlined by barium trickling between the intussusceptum and the outer wall, giving the "coiled spring effect" common in this entity.

tumors, especially lymphomas, may present as intussusceptions.[55,56] Therefore, undue force should not be used to reduce the intussusception. Wide resection of the ileocecal area is indicated if a tumor is suspected.

FACTORS IMPORTANT IN POSTOPERATIVE CARE

In the usual case, only routine gastrointestinal decompression by nasogastric tube and adequate fluid and electrolyte support until resumption of oral feedings are required. For the severely ill child, however, maximum postoperative resuscitation may be required, including ventilatory support (see discussion below).

ASSOCIATED ANOMALIES

There are no anomalies associated with this lesion.

PROGNOSIS

Prognosis is generally excellent.

DISCUSSION

This entity should be straightforward to diagnose and to treat. Early diagnosis should mean low morbidity, no mortality, and over 50 percent of patients treated without surgery.[54]

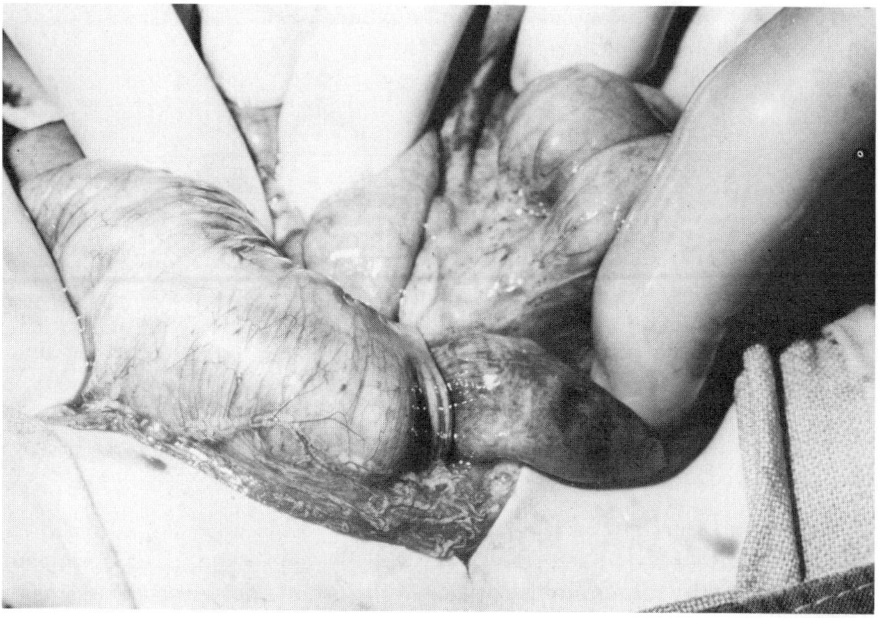

FIG. 50. Operative view of a typical intussusception with the intussusceptum to the right being slowly reduced by backward compression through the outer wall from the left. Hemorrhage in the wall of the intussuscepted bowel is apparent.

Because of delays in diagnosis, this entity frequently requires surgery for nonreduction by hydrostatic barium enema. Delays lead to an unacceptably high incidence of necrotic intestine, requiring resection and resulting in serious postoperative morbidity.

Even when the bowel is viable, reduction of a long-standing intussusception may lead to severe postoperative peritonitis due to loss of integrity of the bowel wall. Some of the most severe cases of sepsis seen in childhood occur in these children. Optimal care with regard to electrolytes and volume replacement, antibiotics, pulmonary support, and perhaps steriods for their controversial role in offsetting the deleterious effects of lysosomal enzymes[57,58] will see most of these children through. Unfortunately, children still die from this basically benign lesion.

In the child over 2 years of age, or when the intussusception recurs, strong suspicion should exist that a lead point is present. Common among these are Meckel's diverticulum, polyps, duplications, and occasionally tumors, especially lymphomas. In the classic age range of infancy, the intussusception is usually "idiopathic" and is thought to be due to hypertrophy of Peyer's patches as a result of systemic viral infections. Recent studies suggest that lead points rarely reduce, so that an attempt at hydrostatic reduction is indicated at all ages and for any number of recurrences.[59] Surgery is indicated only when complete reduction is not achieved.

COLONIC OBSTRUCTIONS

Colonic obstructions include colonic atresia, colonic stenosis, aganglionic megacolon (Hirschsprung's disease), and meconium plug syndrome or small left colon syndrome (SLCS).

USUAL PRESENTATION

Atresia presents with the gradual onset of obstructive symptoms in the newborn period, with distention and eventually emesis and failure to tolerate feedings. Usually meconium is not passed, but this is not invariably the case.

Stenosis may present with symptoms similar to those of atresia or with gradual or intermittent obstructive symptoms. Symptoms may not occur until well beyond the newborn period. Usually meconium is passed.

Aganglionic megacolon, or Hirschsprung's disease, most frequently presents with obstruction in the newborn period but evolving more gradually than in the case of the small or large bowel atresias. Ninety-four percent fail to pass meconium in the first 24 hours,[60] and many appear initially as meconium plug syndrome.[61]

Meconium may be passed, and even transitional or milk stools may follow. Distention and decreased stools or diarrhea then develop, frequently with minimal emesis. Feedings often continue to be tolerated well. However, enterocolitis may develop at any time and present with gray-tan watery diarrhea, dehydration, sepsis, and a rapid downhill course.

Some children with Hirschsprung's disease present minimal symptoms in the newborn or early infancy period and may attain ages well into childhood before the diagnosis is made. They are exceptions, however. In retrospect, even in these youngsters, the stools were usually abnormal from infancy. Most children with Hirschsprung's disease, however, have symptoms, and often severe ones, very early in life.

Meconium plug syndrome and small left colon syndrome are becoming more frequently recognized problems.[62] Clinically, they are usually indistinguishable from meconium ileus, Hirschsprung's disease, and the lower bowel atresias. Failure to pass meconium is the cardinal finding, and gradual abdominal distention and obstructive vomiting are noted over the first few days of life.

These entities are seen with considerably increased frequency in infants of diabetic mothers.[62,63] The diagnosis of meconium plug syndrome or small left colon syndrome should never be fully accepted until meconium ileus (cystic fibrosis) and Hirschsprung's disease are totally ruled out.

DIAGNOSTIC TESTS

Plain X-ray Studies

Abdominal x-rays are the most important initial aides in the differentiation of these entities from higher obstructions. Colonic atresias or stenoses will show air-filled dilated bowel, often with a large loop in the obvious distribution of the large bowel (Fig. 51); so will Hirschsprung's disease (Fig. 52). In meconium plug syndrome and SLCS, films may show bowel suspected to be colon but will also frequently present findings similar to meconium ileus with a disparity of dilatation of the loops, sparse numbers of air-fluid levels, and a soap bubble appearance of air and meconium (see Fig. 47). The bowel dilatation is often less marked than in colonic atresia or Hirschsprung's disease because, as in meconium ileus, the inspissated meconium holds the bowel walls together, preventing full dilatation. Another explanation for this is presented below.

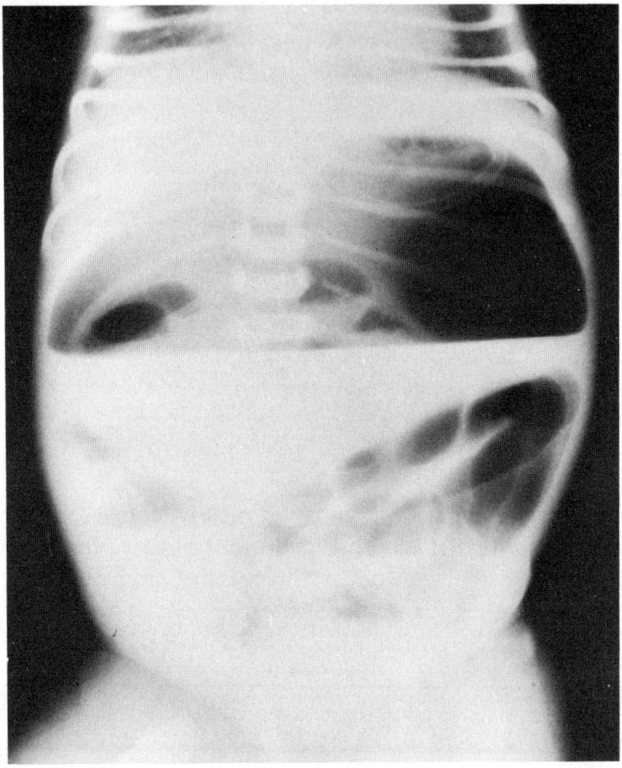

FIG. 51. Very dilated loop of bowel in distribution of transverse colon with air–fluid level traversing entire abdomen. Nasogastric tube decompressing the stomach lessens the likelihood that this is a large dilated stomach. A contrast enema study is mandatory to confirm that this is in fact colon and therefore colonic atresia.

Contrast Enema Studies

If Hirschsprung's disease or colonic atresia is suspected, a barium enema should be done initially. This will demonstrate the obstruction in colonic atresia directly, and will often show the transmition zone of Hirschsprung's diasease in the most common sigmoid location. In Hirschsprung's disease an important part of the examination is the postevacuation lateral film of the pelvic colon. Often the view is best 24 hours after the initial examination (Fig. 53). A rectal level transition zone and narrowed distal bowel may be well demonstrated, but in early infancy this may not be clearly recognizable (Fig. 54). Failure to empty the barium in 24 hours is highly suggestive of Hirschsprung's disease.[64]

If there is suspicion of meconium ileus, meconium plug syndrome, or

SLCS, full-strength water-soluble contrast media should be used for the initial study. Complete reflux well into the small bowel must be achieved (Fig. 55). When meconium plug syndrome is present, the plugs are often encountered quite early in the study. What has been differentiated as SLCS often lacks definite plugs. The bowel should be repeatedly filled with contrast material until easy flow ceases, and then emptying should be allowed (Fig. 55, right). With each cycle of filling and emptying, additional plugs or proximal meconium are loosened and evacuated (Fig. 56). Eventually, easy reflux into small bowel loops demonstrates that the obstruction has been relieved.

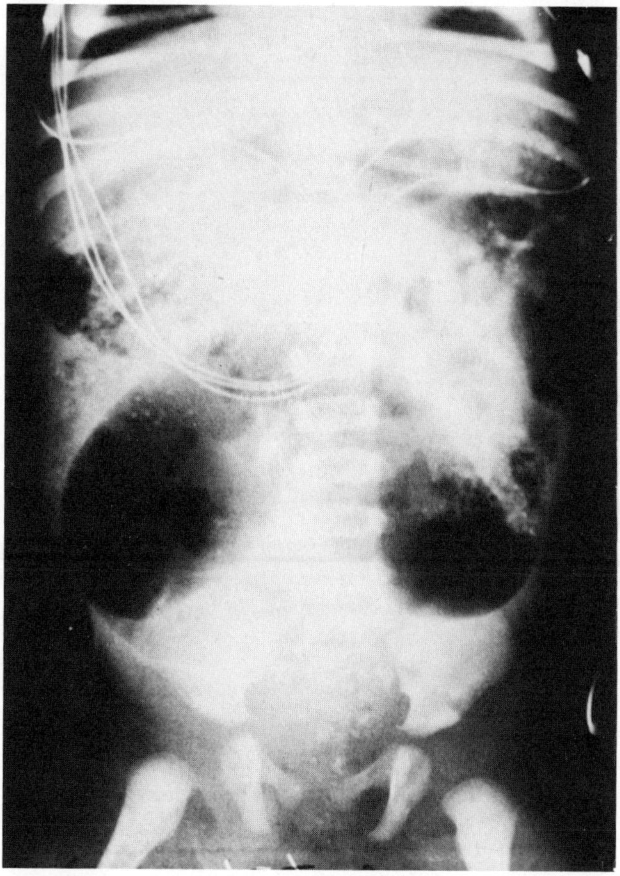

FIG. 52. Abdominal radiograph of large loop of dilated bowel with smaller air shadows scattered throughout abdomen. This is suggestive of but not diagnostic of large bowel obstruction, probably Hirschsprung's disease. Confirmatory barium enema is mandatory.

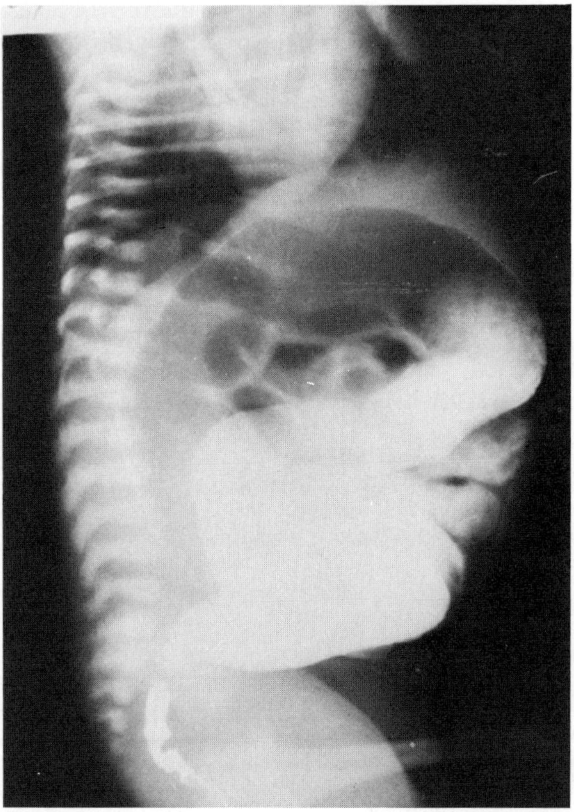

FIG. 53. Classic funnel-shaped transition zone and failure to empty barium on 24-hour postevacuation film of lateral pelvic colon in a patient with Hirschsprung's disease. Unfortunately, this diagnostic picture is infrequently found in the newborn period.

RESUSCITATION AND TRANSPORTATION REQUIREMENTS

Nasogastric tube decompression to prevent reflux and aspiration of gastric contents is all that is usually required.

PROPER HANDLING

The usual procedures for dealing with obstruction should be instituted,

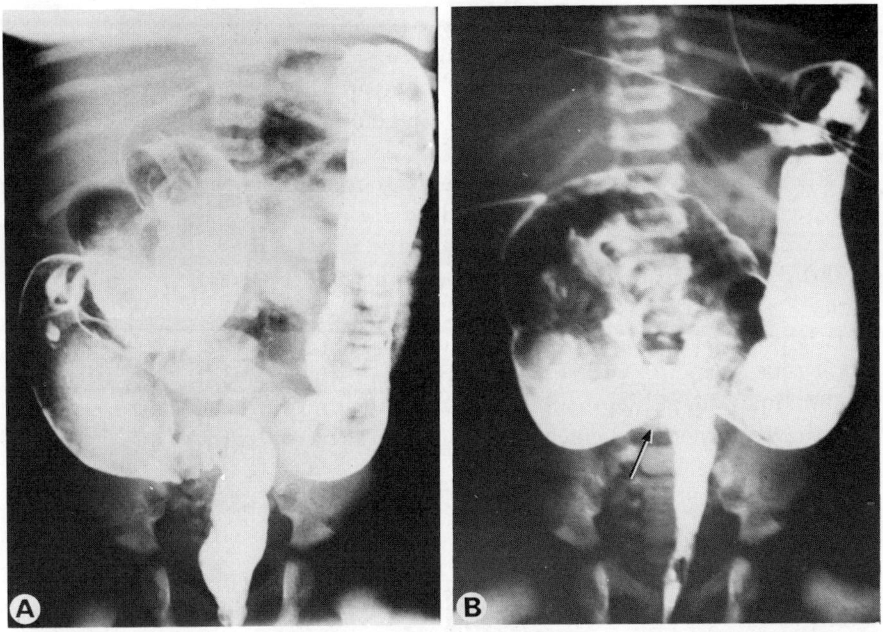

FIG. 54A and B: Views of two separate barium enema studies in a patient with Hirschsprung's disease. Both are early postevacuation films. The change of caliber of the bowel at the distal sigmoid colon can be appreciated. The redundant dilated sigmoid colon courses to the right initially, a not infrequent finding in the newborn infant.

including nasogastric suction to prevent aspiration and the establishment of a good intravenous line for adequate fluid, electrolyte, and nutritional maintenance. Particularly in meconium plug syndrome and SLCS, hypoglycemia must be looked for and corrected.[63] Usually, the proper diagnosis can be established rapidly and corrective measures instituted, allowing early return to normal alimentation so that TPN is rarely indicated.

When water-soluble agents are used for contrast, a secure intravenous line must be established prior to the procedure, and successful entry of contrast into the small bowel should immediately be followed by a push of 20 ml/kg of D_5/RL, preferably with 5 g/100 ml of salt-poor albumin. Following this, continuation of an increased rate of fluid administration should be indicated by urine output; remember, however, that absorption of the dye may temporarily produce an "inappropriate" diuresis. At least a 24-hour careful followup maintaining adequate urine output (40 ml/kg per day) is mandatory.

Even when the dye enters only the large bowel, there may be a large shift of fluid intralumenally, the reason for this being the hyperosmolarity of water-soluble agents (1500 to 2000 mOsm) compared to extracellular fluid osmolarity (approximately 289 mOsm).[45] Therefore, increased intravenous fluid may be required in such instances.

When Hirschsprung's disease is the diagnosis, the threat of enterocolitis is ever present. If it already exists, rapid work-up for sepsis and the institution of broad antibiotic coverage in high dosage may be lifesaving. The general work-up and approach discussed in the chapter on sepsis is completely applicable.

It is essential to provide rapid decompression of the colon. Occasionally, rectal tube washouts will suffice temporarily, if the tube can be passed into the proximal dilated segment. Thorough and continued decompression must be achieved; otherwise, emergency colostomy is mandatory.

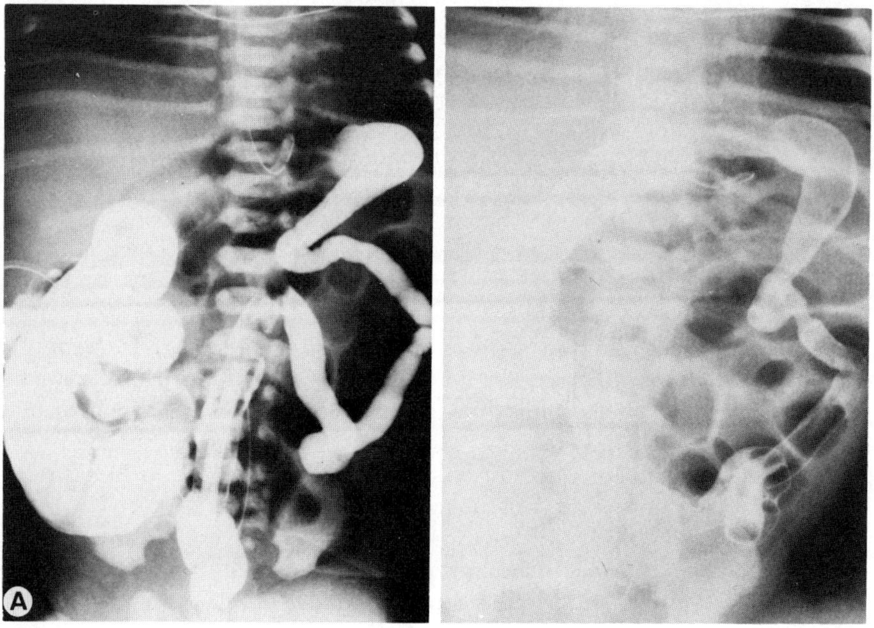

FIG. 55. (A) Water-soluble contrast medium fills small left colon without obvious meconium plugs. The dye has refluxed into dilated proximal bowel loops. (B) Early emptying film shows radiopaque plugs in lumen of left colon.

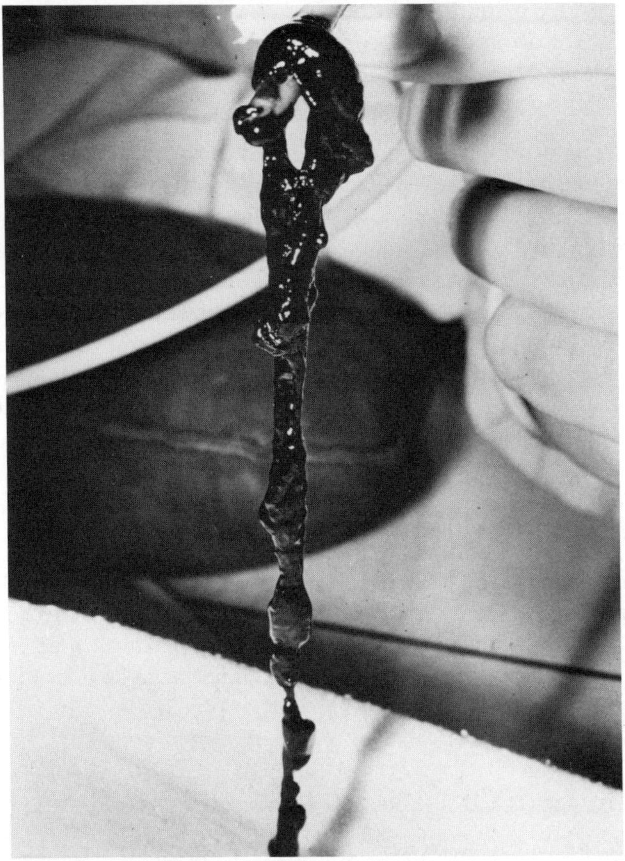

FIG. 56. Part of a long plug or chain of meconium evacuated after water-soluble contrast enema.

CHOICE OF SURGICAL PROCEDURES

Meconium Plug Syndrome and Small Left Colon Syndrome

The water-soluble enema is most often curative, although several attempts may be necessary.

Colonic Atresia or Stenosis

If a localized segment is involved, the segment can be resected and reconstruction with end-to-end anastomosis achieved. Cecostomy may provide some protection to a tenuous or markedly disparate anastomosis.

When the entire distal bowel is atretic or underdeveloped, colostomy with hope of eventual pull-through reconstruction is indicated.

Aganglionic Megacolon

When Hirschsprung's disease is diagnosed in the newborn period, an early colostomy is required to prevent enterocolitis. When the diagnosis is doubtful by x-ray and other causes of obstruction have been ruled out, rectal biopsy will establish or rule out the diagnosis.[65] Once the diagnosis is made with reasonable certainty, colostomy should be done. The placement of the stoma in ganglionated bowel must be confirmed by frozen-section biopsy examination. We prefer to place the colostomy in the most distal ganglionated bowel that can be conveniently looped up to the surface. If rectal biopsy has not been previously performed (ie, when the diagnosis is well established by barium x-ray), a biopsy of the most distal pelvic colon should also be taken to confirm the diagnosis.

Corrective Surgery

Corrective surgical procedures include Swenson endorectal pull-through, the classical procedure;[66] Duhamel posterior coloproctostomy and its modifications;[67—69] and Soave's endorectal pull-through and its modifications. [69—72] Consult a standard text and the referenced articles for details and discussion of these procedures.

FACTORS OF IMPORTANCE IN POSTOPERATIVE CARE

Large bowel surgery in infants requires attention to the details of good fluid, electrolyte, and nutritional management, which are essential for the success of any major surgical procedure. Good mechanical preparation of the bowel is the best safeguard against fecal soilage and infection.

Good colostomy care includes careful attention to the condition of the skin and assurance that an adequate stoma is maintained. Digital or catheter dilatation by the mother combined with frequent checkups and more thorough dilation by the surgeon are important.

ASSOCIATED ANOMALIES

Associated anomalies are rare. The megacystis previously associated with Hirschsprung's disease[73] is now thought to be due to chronic obstruction from fecal impaction and is usually relieved with treatment of the aganglionic colon.

PROGNOSIS

These infants generally do well if properly corrected. Occasionally, incontinence and constipation are problems after surgery for Hirschsprung's disease. These can usually be avoided by careful intraoperative technique and diligent postoperative care including indicated anastomotic dilatations.

A child once having had enterocolitis has an increased risk of having it again even after proper treatment for the underlying lesion. This is especially true if any low-grade obstruction subsequently develops. The reason for this propensity is unclear.

DISCUSSION

Most of the factors of importance have already been elucidated. It is important to grasp the concept thoroughly that a baby presenting with obstruction early in life, whose x-rays show gas well along in the bowel, falls into the group that includes distal small bowel atresias, colon atresias, meconium ileus, meconium plug syndrome, SLCS, and Hirschsprung's disease. The extreme rarity of colon atresia or stenosis places it far down the list for consideration. If dilated bowel following the usual course of the colon can be seen, a large bowel lesion such as "plug," SLCS, or aganglionosis should be suspected. Remember, however, that no definite decision about the level of obstruction should be made on plain x-ray evidence alone, because differentiating large from small bowel in infancy on plain films is subject to great inaccuracy. When a soap bubble appearance consistent with meconium ileus is present, but there appears to be gas present in the colon, meconium plug syndrome or SLCS is most probable. If obviously much dilated gas-filled colon is present, Hirschsprung's disease is most likely.

When no apparent colon pattern is present, the differential is between distal small bowel atresia and meconium ileus. Often the plain films will make the differential, showing "soap bubbles," disparity in the size of the loops, and sparse numbers of air–fluid levels in meconium ileus,[41] with more clearly gas-filled, uniformly dilated loops in atresia.

In any event, a water-soluble contrast enema will make the diagnosis and frequently provide treatment for meconium ileus, meconium plug syndrome, or SLCS. It will confirm distal ileal atresia (see Fig. 6) and may show the transition zone in aganglionosis. Only if Hirschsprung's disease is the most likely diagnosis from the plain films should the first enema study be done with barium.

We have chosen to consider meconium plug syndrome and small left colon syndrome as variations of the same entity. Meconium plug syndrome was first described by Clatworthy in 1956.[74] The etiology was never defined but was generally ascribed to the consistency of the meconium. No abnormalities of the meconium have ever been demonstrated.[75] The narrow caliber of the bowel was ignored. Many denied the existence of meconium plug syndrome as a real entity. Others lumped all non-Hirschsprung's colonic obstructions under this diagnosis. Gradually, it became obvious that the entity occurred most frequently in infants of diabetic mothers.

Recently, several authors have separated off a group of patients from meconium plug syndrome in whom the plugs are less obvious and the caliber change in the bowel occurs at or near the splenic flexure. They have named this the small left colon syndrome.[62,63] Much interesting speculation and some investigation have ensued regarding the etiology of this lesion. Philippart,[63] who limits application of this diagnosis (SLCS) specifically to infants of diabetic mothers, has pointed to the elevation of glucagon in the hypoglycemic infant and directed attention to work done by Kock and others[76] suggesting that glucagon may produce a spastic type of ileus in the sigmoid colon.

Further investigations may clarify the etiologies of these entities. For the present, however, the following points are important and applicable to both lesions:

1. This entity is real and produces total or partial obstruction.
2. If unrelieved, necrosis and perforation of the proximal bowel can occur. There should be a sense of urgency about treatment.
3. These infants can be relieved by water-soluble contrast enemas. Repeated enemas should be given until the obstruction is clearly relieved.
4. Hirschsprung's disease may be the underlying etiology, especially in infants of nondiabetic mothers. Follow-up barium studies should be done at once if the baby fails to establish a normal defecation pattern after the initial obstruction has been relieved.[61]
5. If a normal pattern seems to be established, we have insisted on a follow-up barium enema at 4 weeks of age to avoid missing Hirschsprung's disease.
6. Although barium enema may relieve the obstruction in these entities, it may fail to do so. Certainly the water-soluble agents work better. We have seen three infants in whom barium failed to relieve the obstruction. One of these perforated. Others have had similar experiences.

The continued use of water-soluble agents has been questioned on three grounds.[44,45,61]

1. They produce hypovolemia by creating an osmotic gradient that draws large volumes of body fluid into the lumen of the bowel.[44] This is part of the reason for their success. This hypovolemic effect must be countered by adequate isotonic intravenous fluid administration.

2. The specific agent most widely used, Gastrografin, contains Tween 80.[45] This has been implicated as the cause of an enterocolitis-like picture with perforation in a small number of cases. Similar contrast agents without Tween 80 have not produced this problem clinically or in the laboratory.[45,46]

3. Poole and Rowe have pointed out that the use of water-soluble contrast enemas for distal bowel obstructions may risk missing an infant with Hirschsprung's disease.[61] Failure to empty a barium enema has been an important signal that Hirschsprung's disease is present. The water-soluble agent may be emptied by the aganglionic bowel, delaying the diagnosis. This point is extremely important, and we have therefore insisted for some time now that any child with meconium plug syndrome or SLCS have very careful follow-up. If the child's stool pattern is normal we have reevaluated him at 1 month of age with screening plain films and barium enema if indicated. At any time that the stool pattern is abnormal, a barium enema has then been done.

We would therefore advise using a hyperosmolar agent without Tween 80 as the first choice for these enema studies, unless Hirschsprung's disease is the suspected diagnosis. If this proves to be unsuccessful in reaching bowel proximal to the obstruction, a repeat attempt with Tween 80 would be indicated. This is less likely to be necessary in meconium plug syndrome or SLCS than in meconium ileus with its intrinsically abnormal tenacious meconium.

Properly applied with adequate protection against the hypovolemic effect, these agents have relieved obstruction for innumerable infants without complications. They have enabled infants with cystic fibrosis to have their bowel obstructions relieved without surgery, avoiding the risk of anesthesia in these infants with their high susceptibility to pulmonary complications. These agents should not be banished,[44,61] but as with all therapeutic modalities they must be applied with knowledge and attention to detail.

IMPERFORATE ANUS

This category includes imperforate anus, covered anus, anorectal atresias, and the very rare rectal atresias and stenoses.

USUAL PRESENTATION

Invariably, a normal anus is not found in the usual location. A fistula may be present at birth or may develop subsequently. Meconium passage depends on the presence or absence of a fistula. The infant gradually becomes distended and eventually develops a full picture of bowel obstruction if no fistula is present.

DIAGNOSTIC TESTS

A thorough examination of the perineum, noting the character and position of any stomas, should be performed. In the female infant, a fistula should be sought for carefully, especially in the posterior vulvar fourchette. Gentle probing of this area with a small-caliber soft rubber or plastic catheter may demonstrate the opening. Force should not be applied to the catheter, and metal instruments should be avoided (Fig. 57).

Upside-down lateral x-rays of the pelvic colon have classically been used to determine the level of the bowel relative to the puborectalis sling.[77] They are dependable only after 24 hours and after at least 20 minutes of holding the baby upside down to ensure that the gas has reached the end of the bowel. If an external fistula is present these films are unnecessary. Early plain abdominal x-rays should be obtained to rule out concomitant duodenal atresia.

If a late perineal fistula develops or if any forceful manipulation or probing has been used to produce fistulization, injection of contrast material into the resulting tract is essential to define the anatomy.

RESUSCITATION AND TRANSPORTATION REQUIREMENTS

The inexperienced referring physician should be urged not to probe or puncture any perineal area suggestive of a fistula, unless meconium is passing from it spontaneously. Nasogastric tube decompression should be provided during transport.

PROPER HANDLING

The goal in managing an infant with imperforate anus is to define the exact relationship of the bowel to the puborectalis sling mechanism. This sling, which enwraps the distal rectum, is the most important factor in fecal continence.[78] The external sphincter is of secondary importance, and is much overemphasized in most discussions of this lesion.

Before any definitive operative maneuver is attempted, this relationship must be unequivocally defined. If this proves to be impossible in the neonatal period, a colostomy should be performed to relieve the obstruction and allow time for careful subsequent evaluation.

Basically, there are three anatomic variations of anorectal atresia:

1. The low type, in which the bowel has traversed, and is properly enwrapped by, the puborectalis sling
2. An intermediate type, in which the termination of the bowel is at the level of the sling and exact definition is difficult preoperatively
3. The high type, in which the bowel is clearly above the level of the sling and requires more extensive surgical correction to achieve the normal relationships

When a fistula is present, the level of the bowel can be reliably defined. An external fistula is associated with a low-type atresia. Thus, in the male any opening on the perineum or along the scrotal raphe may be assumed to be associated with a bowel that has traversed the puborectalis sling. In the female, external-type fistulas present on the perineum and in the vulvar fourchette. Low vaginal fistulas may also be associated with bowel that has traversed the sling, but Stephens warns that these are equivocal and that errors may result.[78]

When no fistula is present, but radiographs suggest a fairly low lesion, a

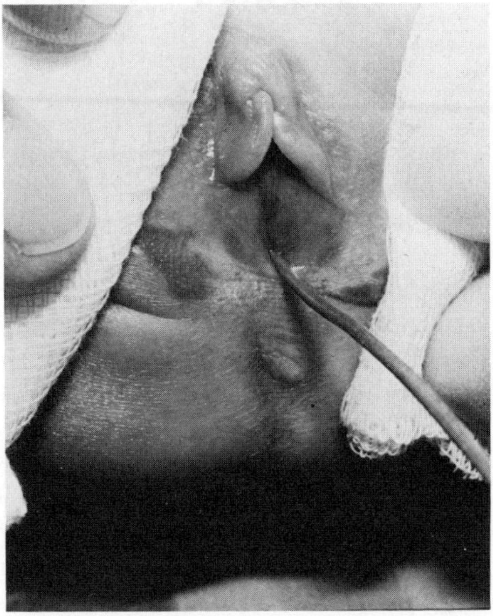

FIG. 57. Perineum of a female infant with imperforate anus. A soft rubber catheter is inserted into the fistula in the vulvar fourchette.

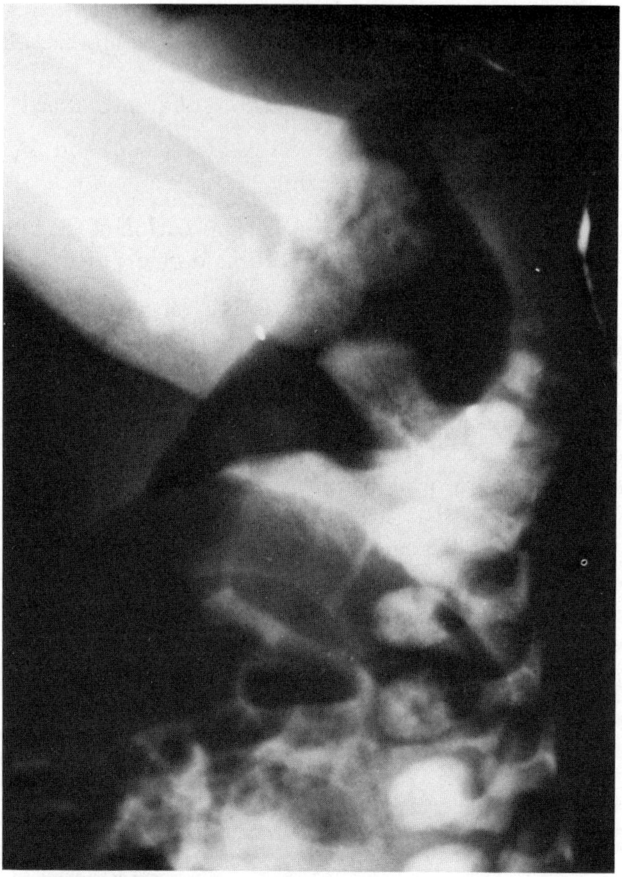

FIG. 58. Lateral radiograph of infant held upside down for 15 to 20 minutes. The rectal air shadow approaches to within a few millimeters of the perineal marker, suggesting a low-type imperforate anus.

period of observation of 24 to 48 hours is warranted (Fig. 58). A definite fistula tract may become obvious during this period[79] (Fig. 59). The infant should be supported with nasogastric tube decompression, intravenous fluids and calories, and antibiotics during this time.

If no fistula develops, carefully performed upside-down roentgen studies should be performed to determine the relationship of the apparent termination of the bowel represented by the end of the air column to the perineum and bony landmarks.[77] Interpretation by a knowledgeable pediatric radiologist is essential at this point. A cystogram and voiding cystourethrogram will help to define an occult rectourethral fistula in a male. Dorsal angulation or "beaking" of the urethra suggests a fistulous attachment.[78] Such a fistula should make colostomy and subsequent sacroperineal repair mandatory. The guiding principle for treatment of the lesion must always be: if in doubt, perform a colostomy in the newborn period.

CHOICE OF SURGICAL PROCEDURES

Depending on the results of the period of observation and the roentgen evaluation, the following choices are available:

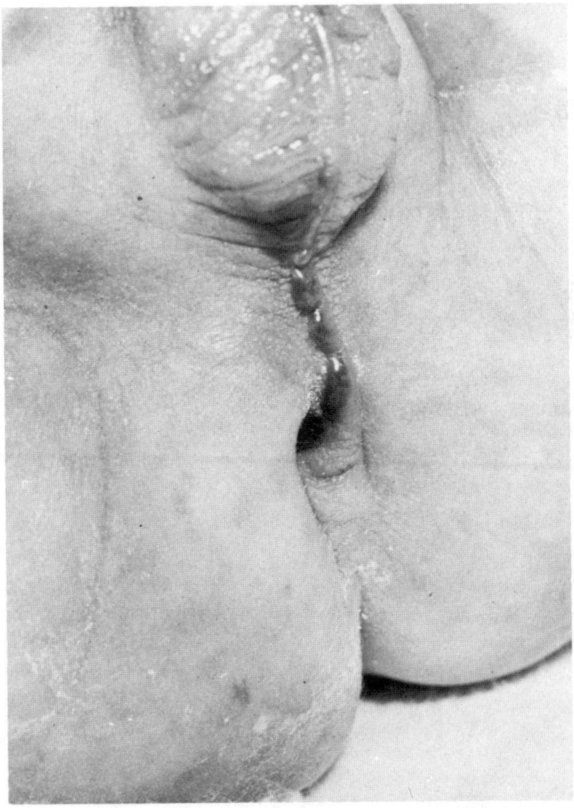

FIG. 59. Twenty-four hours after the inverted radiograph in Figure 58, beads of meconium can be seen coursing along the scrotal raphe, confirming a perineal fistula and a low-type imperforate anus.

1. Low type
   a. Rupture a covered anal membrane.
   b. Dilate the fistula and delay perineal anoplasty for 3 to 4 months (Fig. 60).
   c. Proceed with a perineal anoplasty in the neonatal period.
2. Intermediate type
   a. If a fistula is present that can be dilated, dilate and perform sacroperineal pull-through at 9 to 12 months. This usually applies only to a female infant with a low vaginal fistula.
   b. If no fistula is present, perform a colostomy and delay sacroperineal pull-through until 9 to 12 months.

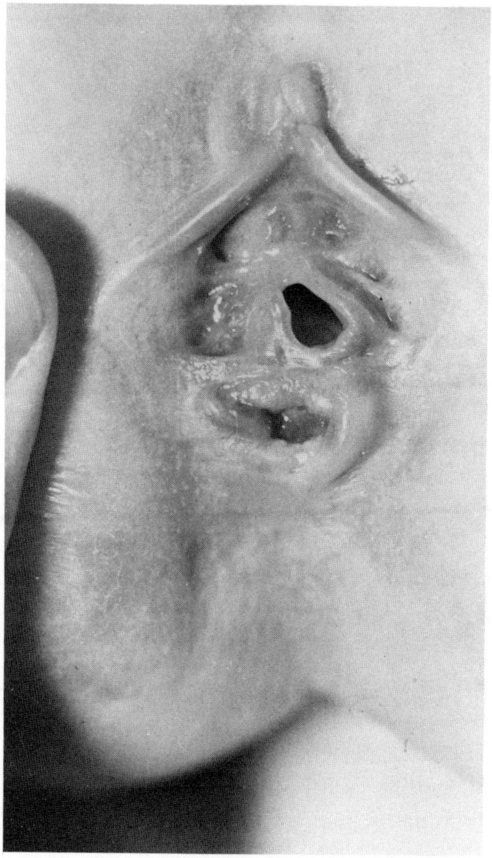

FIG. 60. Female infant perineum with low-type imperforate anus with anoperineal fistula just behind the vulva.

3. High type: all of these lesions will require colostomy followed by sacroperineal or abdominal sacroperineal pull-through at 9 to 12 months.

Stephens demonstrated the value of the sacral approach for identifying the puborectalis muscle sling and ensuring that the pulled-through bowel passes through it properly.[78] This procedure is easier to perform in a larger baby. It is for this reason that a colostomy is performed initially in all lesions other than the clearly defined low type. The definitive pull-through procedure is then performed when the infant weighs 18 to 20 pounds, which is usually around 9 to 12 months of age.

FACTORS OF IMPORTANCE IN POSTOPERATIVE CARE

Regardless of the stoma provided for temporary or permanent defecation, it must be dilated as needed to keep it adequately open and functioning. Providing the mother with the means to do this either with her finger, a catheter, or an appropriate dilator is helpful. The stoma should be checked regularly by the surgeon to ensure proper size and functioning.

ASSOCIATED ANOMALIES

Including the rectourinary fistulas, there is a 40 percent associated renal tract anomaly rate, and repeated intravenous pyelograms are indicated until the normality of the genitourinary tract is reliably established. Duodenal atresia and esophageal atresia are associated with greater than a random incidence.[29]

PROGNOSIS

In the usual case, without other life-threatening anomalies, prognosis for survival is excellent. The long-term question is one of fecal continence, and this is dependent on the intactness of the innervation, the correctness of the surgical repair, and the subsequent functional ability of the child.

DISCUSSION

As discussed above, the most important factor in the newborn period is to avoid the wrong surgical procedure, inflicting irrevocable damage on the anoperineal tissues. Familiarity with the types and classification of anorectal anomalies is important,[80] but, in general, the safest guideline is that a low-type fistula such as a perineal or vestibulofourchette indicates a low lesion that can be treated transperineally, and a high-type fistula, or absence of a fistula, indicates a high-type lesion that should be treated with colostomy in the newborn period.

The most important consideration is the relationship of the rectum to the puborectalis sling mechanism. In high-type lesions, the bowel has not passed through the sling, and great care must be used in handling the sling and placing the bowel through it properly. This is best done through a sacral approach. In the low-type lesions, on the other hand, the bowel has already traversed the sling, and there remains only the need to establish proper communication to the anal area transperineally.

In the intermediate lesions, it is very difficult to be certain of the bowel's relationship to the sling preoperatively, and it is generally safer to utilize the transsacral approach to ensure proper passage of the bowel through the sling. This requires a colostomy in the newborn period and delay of the definitive procedure until 9 to 12 months of age. At all times, great care must be taken to avoid damaging the urinary tract, especially when dealing with a colourethral or rectourethral fistula.

HYDROMETROCOLPOS

This is an unusual anomaly that can be very confusing if never seen previously. It encompasses a range of defects including imperforate hymen, hydrometrocolpos with urogenital sinus, imperforate anus with hydrometrocolpos, and urethrovaginal and rectovaginal fistulas.

USUAL PRESENTATION

This varies with the extent of the anomaly. The most complex and confusing variant is the imperforate anus with hydrometrocolpos, vaginal agenesis, urogenital sinus, and urethrovaginal and rectovaginal fistulas. This baby presents with an abnormal perineum, failure to pass urine and meconium, and usually a distended abdomen and a large abdominal mass.

When only imperforate hymen or vaginal agenesis is present, a neonatal mass may or may not be present. Often, imperforate hymen is asymptomatic until the menarche. On the other hand, when a urethrovaginal fistula is present, the buildup of urine in the vagina produces an enlarging mass, which is the hydrometrocolpos. When accompanied by imperforate anus, signs and symptoms of obstruction of the gastrointestinal tract eventually supervene.

DIAGNOSTIC TESTS

The rest of this discussion applies primarily to the extreme form of this lesion, with rectovaginal and urethrovaginal fistulas, vaginal atresia, and hydrometrocolpos.

If the lesion is suspected on perineal exam, passage of a small, soft, rubber catheter into the urogenital sinus often results in efflux of a large volume of cloudy fluid containing urine, cervical mucus, and meconium (Fig. 61).

Plain abdominal films usually show a large mass rising from the pelvis with the bowel pushed up under the liver and diaphragm.

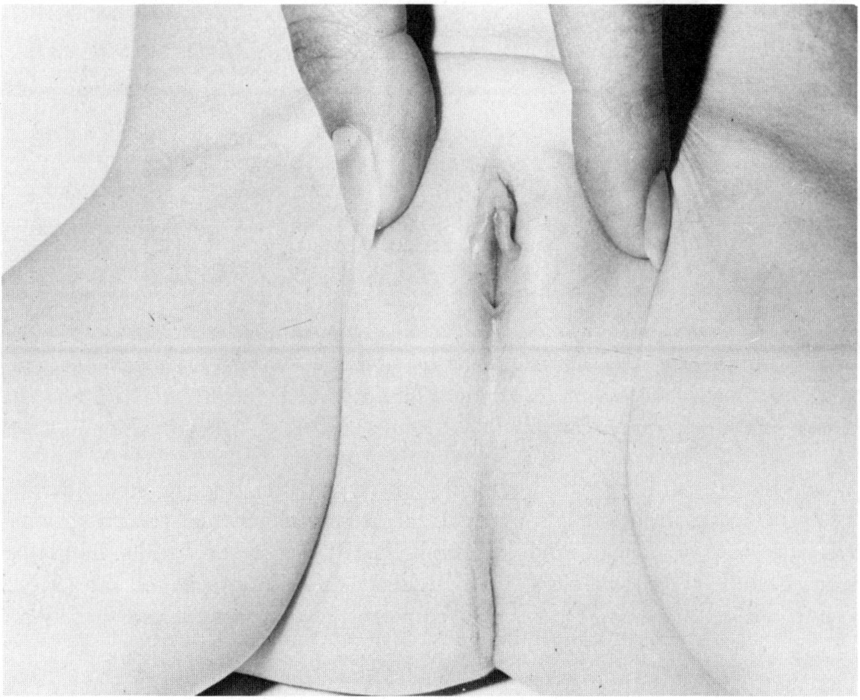

FIG. 61. Infant with hydrometrocolpos, vaginal atresia, rectovaginal fistula, and urethrovaginal fistula. Only one stoma is present on the perineum. This is a urogenital sinus.

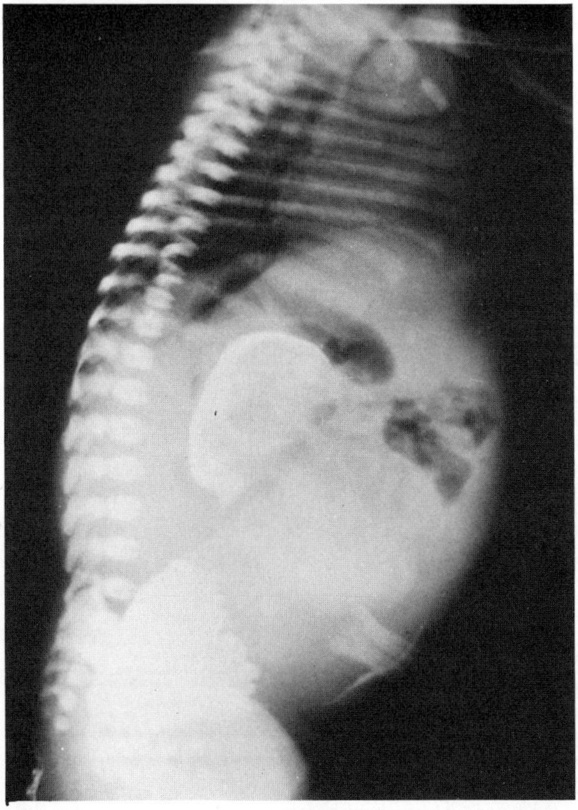

FIG. 62. Infant with hydrometrocolpos. Dye injected into the urogenital sinus outlines the huge hydrocolpos and illustrates the septum within it. The distal colorectum tapers to a fistulous entry into the vagina. This dye was previously injected through a catheter in the rectovaginal fistula.

Dye injected through the perineal catheter will outline the structure that the catheter has entered. If it enters the rectovaginal fistula, the large bowel will be seen to be pushed up out of the pelvis. If the urethrovaginal fistula has been entered, the bladder will fill. If the catheter remains in the vagina, the colpos will be outlined. The fistulas from urethra and rectum may or may not fill concomitantly (Fig. 62).

RESUSCITATION AND TRANSPORTATION REQUIREMENTS

The referring physician is usually confused by this patient. Basically, he recognizes a baby born with marked abdominal distention and an imperforate anus. Usually, nasogastric tube decompression is the only requirement for safe transport to a neonatal center.

PROPER HANDLING

If decompression is achieved by means of the perineal catheter, emergency surgery is obviated. However, successful decompression of the bowel is rarely achieved by this route, so that early colostomy is usually required. Antibiotic coverage is essential with all these fistulous connections.

Early evaluation of urinary function to assess any injury to the kidneys from the low-grade urethral obstruction is mandatory. An early intravenous pyelogram may solve the problem, frequently revealing a moderate degree of obstructive hydroureter and hydronephrosis (Fig. 63). This will usually improve after decompression.

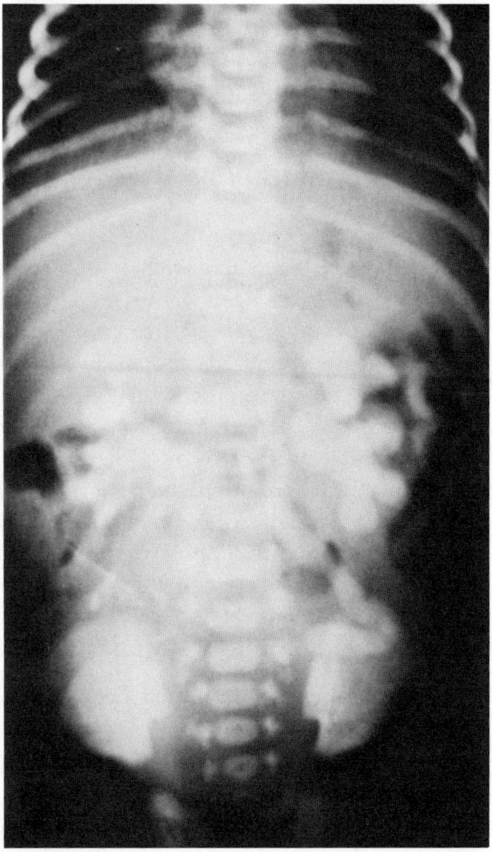

FIG. 63. Intravenous pyelogram on patient with hydrometrocolpos showing hydroureters and hydronephrosis caused by extrinsic obstruction from the large pelvic mass. Resolution of this urinary tract pathology after decompression of the mass should be confirmed by intravenous pyelograms.

If an intravenous pyelogram fails to visualize, the BUN and creatinine should be followed and the intravenous pyelogram repeated in a week or two. A rising BUN indicates obvious renal impairment. If the urinary tract fails to improve, evaluation and correction of any intrinsic urinary tract anomaly should be accomplished before severe renal damage results.

CHOICE OF SURGICAL PROCEDURES

Early exploratory laparotomy with diversion of the bowel from the vagina and establishment of an end colostomy relieves the intestinal obstruction. At that time, if a catheter can be, or has been, easily passed transperineally into the bladder, the urinary tract can probably be decompressed from below.

Inability to decompress the vagina and bladder transperineally requires establishment of a suprapubic cystostomy and usually a tube decompression of the hydrocolpos (Fig. 64). Subsequently, reconstruction of the intestinal tract and vagina will require abdominal sacroperineal pull-through of the colorectum and vaginal pull-through as outlined by Ramenofsky and Raffensperger.[81] The ideal age for this is probably about 9 to 12 months.

FACTORS OF IMPORTANCE IN POSTOPERATIVE CARE

Once the colostomy is established, if transperineal decompression of the hydrocolpos has been achieved, it is very important to maintain this decompression so that free egress of urine is possible. Buildup of urine and cervical secretions in the vagina leads to recurrent infections.

Usually, after a few days of indwelling catheterization, adequate decompression can be maintained without the catheter. However, it is probably wise to instruct the parents in the catheterization technique and have them check the baby once daily by catheterizing the urogenital sinus.

Careful follow-up of the urinary tract function is important, and repeated intravenous pyelograms at three- to four-month intervals should be done to ensure that the hydronephrosis is improving.

ASSOCIATED ANOMALIES

No consistent association has been found.

PROGNOSIS

If the kidneys have not been severely damaged by the prolonged obstruction, and usually they have not, the prognosis for survival is quite good. The

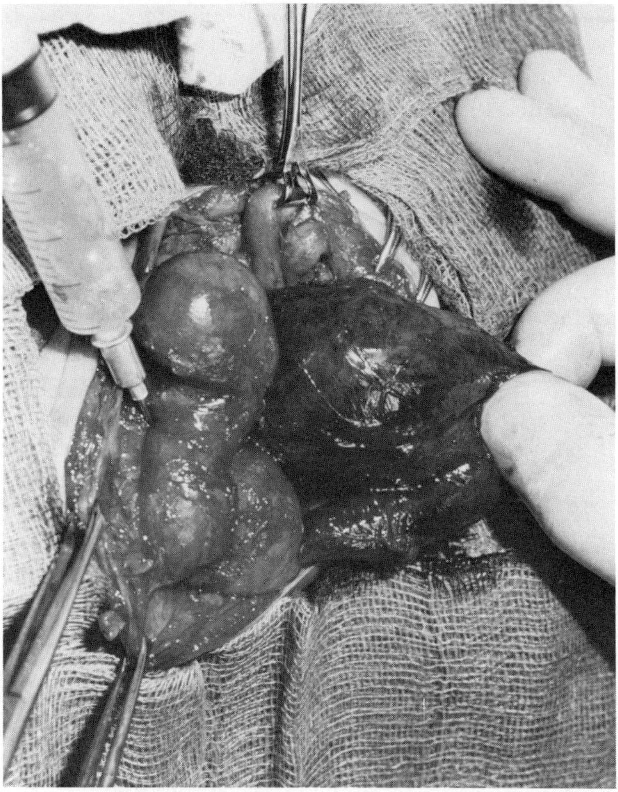

FIG. 64. Initial operative exploration of infant with hydrometrocolpos. Dilated colorectum enters vagina as fistula from the right. The syringe is aspirating cloudy fluid from the hydrocolpos.

prognosis for reconstruction of the anorectum with normal function must be quite guarded, however, since abnormalities of the sling musculature and innervation may be present. Reconstruction of the vagina is readily done, and Raffensperger's approach obviates the problem of damage to the urethral sphincter mechanisms.

DISCUSSION

This is a rare entity which can be quite confusing when seen for the first time. Early recognition and correct initial care can prevent unneeded surgical procedures and damage to vital structures. It should be suspected whenever a child presents with imperforate anus and ambiguous external genitalia, especially if by physical exam or x-ray a mass arising from the pelvis is suspected. Since fusion of part or all of the labia may accompany this entity, the incorrect diagnosis of adrenogenital abnormalities or feminizing tumors may be made. Careful examination including a sinogram usually will at least begin to clarify the situation.

MECONIUM PERITONITIS: IN UTERO PERFORATION OF THE BOWEL

This entity represents perforation of the bowel in utero. Intestinal contents have spilled into the peritoneal cavity, resulting in intraperitoneal calcifications. The perforation subsequently may have healed, leaving an intact bowel; it may remain open, resulting in further postuterine soilage of the peritoneal cavity; or an etiologic atresia with obstruction may persist.[82]

USUAL PRESENTATION

These infants frequently present with a distended edematous abdominal wall. Discoloration of the abdominal wall with a prominent venous pattern is common. The infant may or may not pass meconium. Signs of intestinal obstruction will develop if atresia or meconium ileus is the etiology of the perforation. Acrocyanosis and edema of the extremities are often present.

DIAGNOSTIC TESTS

Plain films of the abdomen may show intraperitoneal calcifications, free air, obstructed loops, and/or ascites.

RESUSCITATION AND TRANSPORTATION REQUIREMENTS

This is another entity that is very confusing to the physician if not previously seen. Nasogastric decompression is the only special requirement.

PROPER HANDLING

Careful evaluation of plain films determines further work-up:

1. If free air is present, urgent surgery is mandatory, and further x-ray work-up is unnecessary.
2. If an obstructive pattern is present, without free air, a rapid evaluation to determine the site and cause of obstruction is warranted. A water-soluble contrast enema may be helpful, especially for meconium ileus.
3. If only intraperitoneal calcifications and/or ascites are present, with a normal intestinal gas pattern all the way to the rectum, a healed perforation may be the diagnosis, and surgery may be unnecessary. The bowel gas should be followed by plain films until either a site of obstruction, free air, or complete continuity of the intestinal tract is demonstrated (Fig. 65).

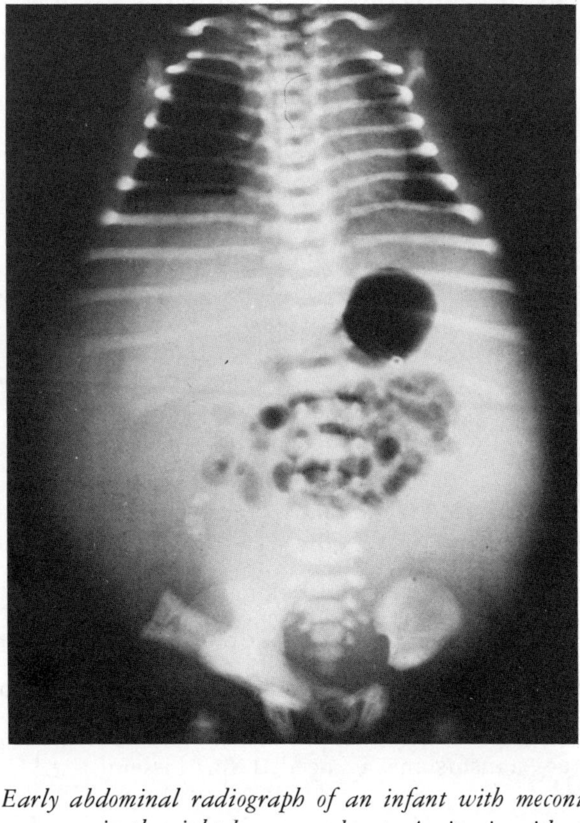

FIG. 65. Early abdominal radiograph of an infant with meconium peritonitis. Calcifications are seen in the right lower quadrant. Ascites is evident throughout the abdomen. The bowel pattern continued to prove normal all the way to the anus, and no surgical procedure was required.

Regardless of the variation of this entity, careful fluid, electrolyte, and nutritional management together with effective antibiotic coverage are essential. A well-functioning intravenous line must be established, and adequate doses of broad-spectrum antibiotics must be given intravenously. These children have an increased risk of developing peritonitis whether or not persistent free perforation is present. Baseline and follow-up cultures should be done.

Because peritonitis is almost surely present on a chemical basis, even in the absence of persisting free perforation, one should expect a fairly large fluid requirement for losses into the bowel and peritoneal cavity.

CHOICE OF SURGICAL PROCEDURES

Once free air or obstruction is demonstrated, surgery must be accomplished as soon as adequate fluids and antibiotics are given and blood is ready. The procedures vary with the cause of obstruction and/or perforation. Although extensive corrective surgical procedures are unwarranted under these conditions, atresias should be treated in the usual fashion with resections and end-to-end primary anastomosis if possible.

Associated meconium ileus is best handled with the Bishop–Koop type of ileoileostomy,[47] unless intraoperative decompression by transrectal washouts can be achieved and the in utero perforation has healed.

When extensive peritonitis is present with firm adhesions, a simple exteriorization procedure is the safest choice. Obviously, each case must be carefully individualized, and no hard and fast rules are possible.

FACTORS OF IMPORTANCE IN POSTOPERATIVE CARE

1. Good fluid, electrolyte, and nutritional care together with continued antibiotic therapy
2. Total parenteral nutrition for prolonged support
3. Frequent cultures and change of antibiotic coverage as indicated
4. Careful monitoring of platelets and peripheral smear for indications of disseminated intravascular coagulopathy
5. Exchange transfusions as needed for disseminated intravascular coagulopathy[83]
6. Secondary surgical procedures as indicated to restore continuity of the gastrointestinal tract

ASSOCIATED ANOMALIES

Other than the etiologic entity of the perforation, no other anomalies are consistently associated. Cystic fibrosis will be present if meconium ileus was the etiology of the perforation.

PROGNOSIS

The main factor influencing survival is infection. Most of the causes of perforation can be corrected surgically. However, even those babies with an intact gastrointestinal tract may succumb to severe and overwhelming gram-negative infection and disseminated intravascular coagulopathy. The sooner the diagnosis is made and treatment for infection begun, the better the prognosis. Delayed diagnosis or withholding of antibiotics to await signs of infection or culture results may result in a mortality. Because the diagnosis is often delayed, allowing peritonitis and infection to become well established, the mortality from this entity remains unnecessarily high.

DISCUSSION

Once a child with this entity survives the newborn period, he has an increased risk of developing intestinal obstruction and portal venous obstruction secondary to umbilical vein–ductus venosus sepsis with pylephlebitis. This may lead to portal hypertension, splenomegaly, hypersplenism, and, in time, esophageal varices with hemorrhage. These significant complications must be watched for. Unfortunately, they cannot be entirely prevented.

FREE PERFORATION IN THE NEWBORN PERIOD

USUAL PRESENTATION

In contrast to a child with in utero perforation, a child with neonatal perforation usually appears to be normal at birth. The first sign of perforation is usually increasing abdominal distention. Obstructive signs such as emesis and failure to pass meconium are usually absent, at least initially. Absence of liver dullness will be noted on physical examination if sought. Unfortunately, sepsis follows very rapidly, and symptoms such as failure to maintain body temperature, ashen mottled appearance, generalized edema, and petechiae may appear early.

DIAGNOSTIC TESTS

Plain films of the abdomen should include an upright view, on which free air usually will be quite apparent (see Fig. 29). It is important, however, to be able to recognize free air on the recumbent film, as this is the view most frequently obtained routinely, especially in emergency portable studies[84] (see Fig. 30).

A generalized lucency in the right upper quadrant overlying the normally homogeneously opaque liver is diagnostic. Other signs include the thickened bowel walls of peritonitis and the "ghost" appearance of air outlining the outside of the bowel.

RESUSCITATION AND TRANSPORTATION REQUIREMENTS

The rapidity of injury from infection in the newborn period warrants initiation of antibiotic therapy prior to transportation. Stabilization of vital signs, provisions for ventilatory support, and the usual nasogastric tube decompression should all be accomplished as well.

PROPER HANDLING

Once suspected, the diagnosis should be rapidly confirmed by x-ray. If not already in place, a nasogastric tube should be inserted and placed to suction to minimize the leakage of additional air and intestinal contents into the peritoneal cavity.

Rapid preparations for surgery should include establishment of a dependable intravenous route, a fluid and electrolyte "push," cross-matching of blood, and administration of high-dose antibiotics. If respiratory distress from compression of the diaphragm is severe, release of air by needle paracentesis may be required.

CHOICE OF SURGICAL PROCEDURES

Free perforation in the neonatal period can be divided into four subclassifications: (a) those resulting from intrinsic obstruction such as atresias, meconium ileus, or aganglionic megacolon; (b) those due to strangulation such as from malrotation with volvulus; (c) "idiopathic" perforations; and (d) neonatal necrotizing enterocolitis with perforation. Of these, the fourth is the most common and most frequently involves the ileocecal area. More extensive involvement of the bowel is not unusual, however.

The etiology of perforation has been variously attributed in the past to "stress ulceration," hypoxia, and vigorous resuscitation with overdistention of the stomach. The true etiology remains in doubt. Presently, neonatal necrotizing enterocolitis (NEC) is the cause of most newborn perforations. Much work has been done to determine the etiology of this lesion. An extensive discussion of NEC is presented in Section II and immediately following this chapter.

Obviously the surgery performed must be tailored to the findings. Control of the perforation by suture or by resection and anastomosis is essential. Occasionally, exteriorization will prove to be safest but should not be the usual procedure.

When atresias are present, they should be treated with resection and primary reconstruction, if viable bowel is available for anastomosis. Meconium ileus and meconium plug may be treated in the usual ways.

Often only a large rent in the greater curvature of the stomach is found with no distal obstruction. This should be debrided to viable tissue, sutured, and protected by a gastrostomy.

Unlike in utero perforations, the soilage and adhesions are of short duration and can usually be readily cleaned up and dissected. In all cases, assurance of the patency and continuity of the entire gastrointestinal tract is mandatory.

FACTORS OF IMPORTANCE IN POSTOPERATIVE CARE

Once again the primary risk and source of mortality is sepsis. Adequate and appropriate antibiotic coverage before, during, and after surgery should be accompanied by frequent cultures, daily platelet count, and smear analysis for developing sepsis and disseminated intravascular coagulopathy. The usual approach to good fluid and electrolyte and nutritional management must be adhered to. Extensive cardiopulmonary support procedures may be needed. The use of multiple exchange transfusions for refractory sepsis and disseminated intravascular coagulopathy will increase survival.[83]

ASSOCIATED ANOMALIES

Generally, there are no anomalies associated with this lesion.

PROGNOSIS

Again, prognosis depends primarily on the control and treatment of sepsis. Mortality remains high but has improved recently.

DISCUSSION

Early recognition and rapid and correct surgical treatment combined with good postoperative multisystem support and treatment for sepsis may improve the presently high mortality rate.

NEONATAL NECROTIZING ENTEROCOLITIS

Although this entity is discussed in Section 2, Chapter 2, under "Free Perforations of the Gastrointestinal Tract," it is such a common and important disease in present-day pediatric surgery that a thorough discussion of the whole spectrum of its clinical manifestations seems warranted here. Section 2 should be reviewed for its discussion of etiologic factors and pathogenesis.

USUAL PRESENTATION

Necrotizing enterocolitis usually becomes manifest in the first week after birth, often at 3 to 5 days of life. Much later presentations are not rare, however, and occasionally a fulminant picture is already present within 48 hours of birth. Frequently, but not invariably, a stressful event can be identified in the infant's recent past history. Stress includes such occurrences as fetal distress at or prior to delivery, in utero sepsis, late third trimester bleeding, multiple births, and a diabetic mother. Neonatal asphyxia, meconium aspiration, and all degrees of respiratory distress may be inciting events.

Early symptoms and signs include irritability, temperature instability, abdominal distention, regurgitant emesis, loose, seedy stools, and streaks of red blood in the stool. Abdominal distention is the most consistent finding.

As the disease becomes more severe, distention worsens, stools become more bloody, bilious aspirates increase, and sepsis is heralded by apnea, bradycardia, hypothermia, and peripheral mottling.

Bowel necrosis, abscess formation, or perforation is indicated by signs of peritonitis. These include edema and hyperemia of the abdominal wall, obvious tenderness to palpation, and occasionally a definite intraperitoneal mass.

DIAGNOSTIC TESTS

Stools should be tested for blood. A nasogastric tube should be passed, aspirated, and placed to intermittent suction. The character of the aspirate should be noted. Plain abdominal radiographs will show a "dirty," mottled bowel pattern with some distention of the bowel loops. Usually the bowel walls are thickened, indicating edema and peritonitis. The cardinal sign of NEC is intramural air or pneumatosis intestinalis. When this is present on the radiographs, the diagnosis is confirmed. Air in the portal venous system is seen in a small number of these patients and is probably indicative of a severe case (Fig. 66). Contrast studies of the bowel are not helpful, and contrast enema is contraindicated in the presence of impending perforation.

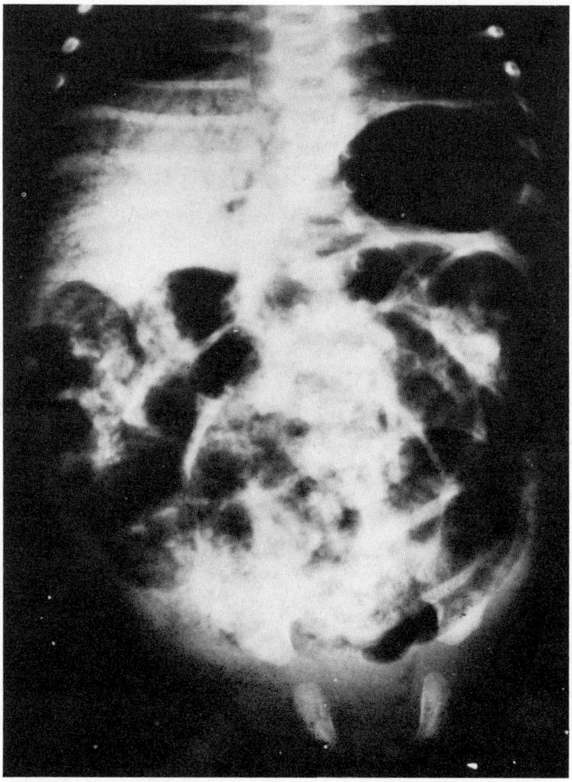

FIG. 66. Abdominal radiograph of infant with neonatal necrotizing enterocolitis. Portal vein gas is evident over the liver. The loops of bowel exhibit a typical mottled or "dirty" appearance. Pneumatosis is probably present in the loops in the high right upper and low left lower quadrants.

RESUSCITATION AND TRANSPORTATION REQUIREMENTS

A nasogastric tube should be in place. If possible, an intravenous line for fluid and antibiotic administration should be established. The baby must be stabilized before and during transport, especially if he is already septic and exhibiting apnea and bradycardia.

PROPER HANDLING

This disease has been devastating in recent years, and the operative mortality has been significant. Children's lives have been saved by surgery before and after necrosis and perforation of the bowel, but far better results are observed when perforation is prevented and the disease responds to medical therapy. It is not known whether there is a fulminant form of the disease which progresses rapidly to necrosis and perforation regardless of therapy. It is clear that most infants respond to medical therapy, avoiding bowel loss and perforation.

Until the natural variations of the disease are more clearly defined, all suspect infants should be placed on a full therapeutic program immediately. This should include (a) complete bowel rest, (b) nasogastric decompression, (c) supportive intravenous fluid and electrolyte therapy, (d) systemic antibiotics with good broad-spectrum, but especially gram-negative, coverage, and (e) cardiovascular and respiratory support as needed. Some feel that intestinal antibiotics given by gastric lavage add an important increment of therapy.[85]

The course of the disease should be monitored by (a) baseline and repeat blood cultures, (b) frequent examination of the abdomen and measurement of its girth, (c) repeated abdominal radiographs to confirm pneumatosis and recognize pneumoperitoneum if perforation supervenes, and (d) continued testing of stools for occult blood.

Although originally surgery was reserved for obvious free perforations or abscess formation at most centers, more recently earlier exploration for signs of peritonitis prior to frank perforation has seemed to result in better survival for these infants.[86]

In addition to those with frank perforation or abscess formation, we have elected to explore babies who, after the establishment of the above medical regimen, have shown any of the following:

1. Edema, hyperemia, and tenderness of the abdomen.
2. Failure to stabilize after 12 to 24 hours of medical treatment. These babies show persistent or newly developed septic signs including temperature instability, apnea, and bradycardia.
3. Presence or evolution of a palpable abdominal mass usually representing an insidious perforation walled off by matted bowel loops.

CHOICE OF SURGICAL PROCEDURES

Many have advocated unequivocally that only proximal enterostomies and resections without anastomoses be done.[87] In general this is a preferable approach, but there are infants whose disease is adequately limited so that safe reconstruction can be done. This is especially suitable for lesions higher in the small bowel for which an "ostomy" would be jejunostomy or high ileostomy. Particularly when the operation is accomplished for necrosis and impending perforation without frank soilage from open perforation, primary reconstruction can be safely accomplished in most cases.

In very severe cases, the entire colon may be necrotic,and total abdominal colectomy is necessary. Since the rectum is usually spared, later ileoproctostomy may be possible.

Because of the severe sepsis that is typical of the postoperative course in these patients, we generally place central venous and arterial monitoring catheters at the same operation.

FACTORS OF IMPORTANCE IN POSTOPERATIVE CARE

Total support is often needed by these infants. This may involve respirator therapy with mechanical ventilation and positive airway pressure, oxygen administration in appropriate percentages, and cardiovascular support with pharmacologic agents such as digitalis derivatives, diuretics, and dopamine. Antibiotics appropriate to the gram-negative organisms should be continued in full dosages. Complete bowel rest must be maintained.

When, as is often the case, gram-negative sepsis leads to disseminated intravascular coagulopathy, we have found repeated exchange transfusions to be efficacious.[83] Some infants have required as many as 26 exchange transfusions to stabilize their clotting factors.

ASSOCIATED ANOMALIES

There are no anomalies consistently associated with NEC.

PROGNOSIS

For the infants who respond to initial medical therapy and remain stable, prognosis is excellent. We have treated them for three weeks with bowel rest and antibiotics. Total parenteral nutritional support is added once the initial septic phase has cleared. A small percentage of these infants develop late strictures, usually in the colon, and these require resection and anastomosis.[88-90] This surgery is performed in a relatively stable, uninfected baby, and results have been good.

The infant who perforates usually has a severe septic course postoperatively, and this results in a significant mortality. With intensive therapy for the sepsis including repeated exchange transfusions, more of these infants are now being saved.

We seem to see a hopeful picture in which most infants operated on for the listed indications prior to perforation will have a less severe postoperative course with improved survival.

DISCUSSION

These are basically normal infants with an acquired illness. Survival usually results in a normal life. Therefore, every effort is warranted to try to salvage them. Much progress has been made since the initial recognition of the increasing incidence of this disease only a few years ago.

This is a lesion in which avoidance of the need for surgery almost guarantees survival but where withholding indicated surgery means almost certain death. The hope for the distant future is prevention, but for the immediate future earlier identification of the infant whose course will lead to perforation will improve survival for these sicker infants.

GASTROSCHISIS

Gastroschisis is an entity whose etiology is not well understood. This defect is thought to be due to a failure of development of an abdominal wall somite, allowing the intestine to herniate into the amniotic fluid.[91]

USUAL PRESENTATION

The infant is born with the intestine herniated through a defect in the abdominal wall, usually just to the right of the umbilicus. The umbilical cord has a normal configuration and relationship to the abdominal wall. Usually only the intestines and occasionally the ovary and tube or testicle are eviscerated, the liver being normally situated in the peritoneal cavity. Because the bowel is not covered by peritoneum in utero, it is thickened, foreshortened, and covered with an exudate. This represents an irritative or chemical peritonitis (Fig. 67).

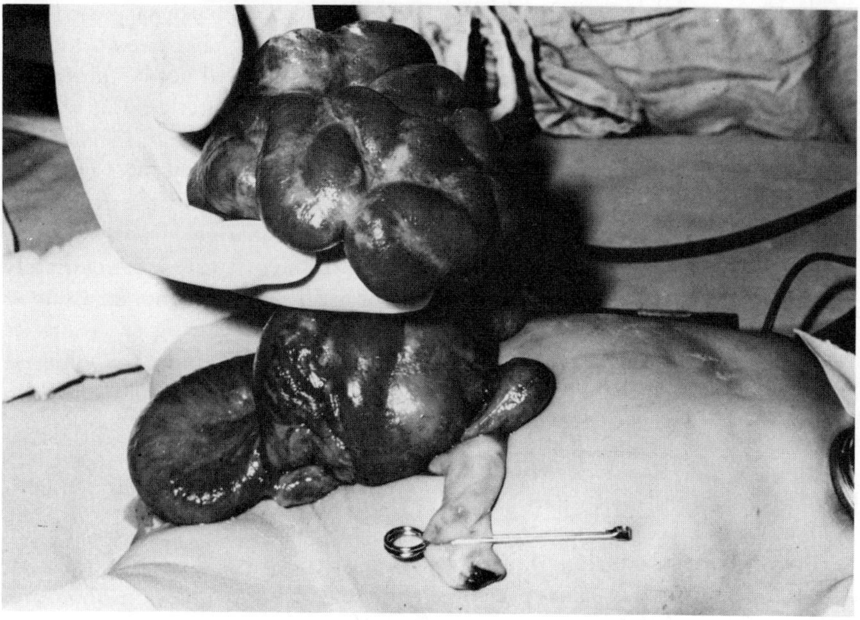

FIG. 67. Infant with gastroschisis. Defect is to right side of umbilical cord, which is flush with the abdominal wall. Note the thickened adherent intestinal loops.

DIAGNOSTIC TESTS

Since the deformity is obvious, no preoperative diagnostic studies are necessary.

RESUSCITATION AND TRANSPORTATION REQUIREMENTS

These infants require early intravenous cannulation and effective volume maintenance. The great surface area of inflamed intestine that is eviscerated and exposed leads to rapid extensive fluid and heat losses with resultant hypovolemic shock and hypothermia. Many of these infants sustain severe ischemic damage to their body tissues from perfusion deficits. A push of 20 ml/kg should be given immediately after cannulation is accomplished. Only D_5/RL or D_5/RL with albumin should be used for resuscitation. Following the push, a rate equal to three to four times the infant's maintenance rate is warranted until the urine output reaches 3 to 5 ml/hour or 40 ml/kg per 24 hours.

The eviscerated bowel should be covered with soft gauze saturated with saline to which a small amount of antiseptic solution* has been added. It should then be supported in such a way that the bowel will not be folded over the edge of the abdominal defect, strangulating its mesenteric blood supply. If the defect is tiny and the mesentery compressed, a 1- to 2-cm incision will widen the defect and loosen the compression. Wrapping the bowel with several turns of soft roller gauze and then girdling this around the trunk in a "figure of eight" fashion will support the bowel adequately.

Broad-spectrum antibiotic coverage should be instituted immediately. Nasogastric tube decompression will prevent aspiration pneumonia. Extra efforts are needed to maintain normal body temperature during the resuscitation efforts and transport. Expeditious transportation should be achieved. Transport should not be delayed if intravenous cannulation is difficult to achieve.

PROPER HANDLING

Any of the resuscitation requirements not accomplished prior to transport should be completed. The patient's state of volume repletion should be evaluated and replacement fluids adjusted appropriately. Normothermia should be maintained or achieved. The condition of the intestines should be checked, and any ischemic obstructions should be relieved. Surgical correction should be scheduled at once.

CHOICE OF SURGICAL PROCEDURES

Whenever possible, primary closure as described by Raffensperger and Jona should be the procedure of choice.[92] This requires experience and sound judgment to select the baby who can tolerate it. It is rarely accomplished as easily as the authors suggest, but, in experienced hands, primary closure is often achieved.

Generally, the limiting factor in any procedure is the degree of interference with respiratory function. The use of mechanical ventilatory assistance for 24 to 48 hours to relieve the infant of extra respiratory work necessitated by a tight closure is acceptable, but the need for markedly increased ventilatory pressures should lead to abandonment of primary closure in favor of a prosthetic pouch.

The technique of Raffensperger and Jona requires the following steps:

*Betadine solution, Purdue Frederick Co., Norwalk, Conn.

1. Washing out of the meconium from the distal bowel with saline enemas
2. Vigorous stretching of the walls of the peritoneal cavity bilaterally from the vertebral column to the edges of the defect
3. Careful dissection and lysis of adhesions among the bowel loops
4. Careful repositioning of the freed intestinal loops into all areas of the abdominal cavity

Step 3 is the limiting factor. If the adhesions are so thick and fibrous that dissection leads to mural damage and extensive hemorrhage, the procedure should be abandoned.

The next best procedure is to perform as much of the procedure for primary closure as is possible and then apply a prosthetic pouch of Silon* (Dacron covered with Silastic*) for gradual reduction of the evisceration[93-95] (Fig. 68).

There probably is no satisfactory third choice. Specifically, skin coverage alone is usually unacceptable.

FACTORS OF IMPORTANCE IN POSTOPERATIVE CARE

1. Continue antibiotic coverage.
2. Achieve complete closure as rapidly as possible. Seven to ten days should be the goal.
3. Achieve and maintain full volume restoration.
4. Monitor arterial blood gases and central venous pressure. Transposition of the umbilical artery[96] and percutaneous cannulation of the superior vena cava from the subclavian vein[97] will facilitate this monitoring (see Section 1, Chapter 3).
5. Recognize sepsis early by platelet count monitoring and frequent blood cultures, and treat it vigorously if it occurs. Repeated exchange transfusions may be needed if overwhelming gram-negative sepsis and disseminated intravascular coagulopathy develop.[83]
6. Initiate central TPN as soon as the need for central venous pressure

*Silastic sheeting, Dow-Corning Corporation, Midland, Mich.

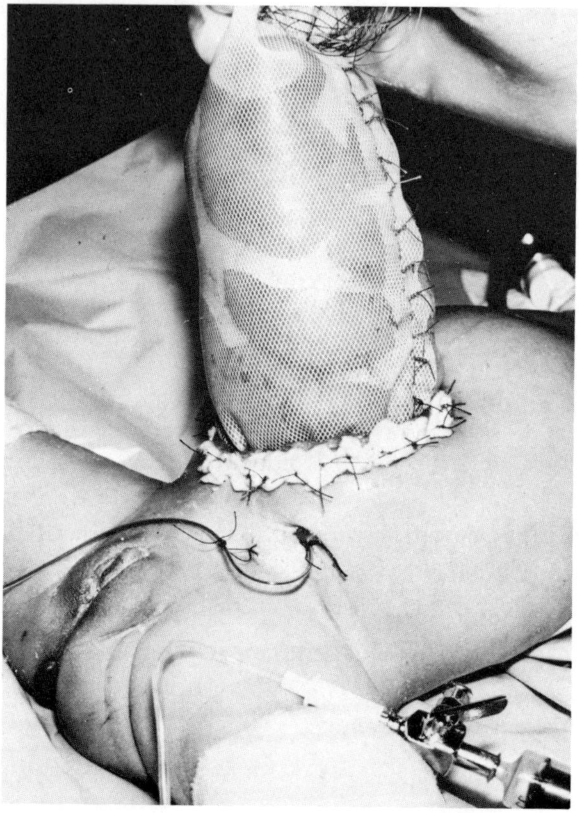

FIG. 68. Gastroschisis treated with Silon pouch technique. Note bolstering of suture line with Teflon felt pledgets. The umbilical artery has been transposed to the left lower abdomen and catheterized for postoperative monitoring of arterial blood gases. (From Filston and Izant, J Pediatr Surg 10:225, 1975)

monitoring has passed. Continue TPN until adequate gastrointestinal feedings are tolerated.[98]

7. Particularly if associated volvulus or atresia has left the infant with a deficient length of intestine, prolonged intolerance of gastrointestinal feedings may be a problem. A program of gradual incremental additions of volume with gradual increases of concentration of predigested formulas should be instituted and maintained until full volumes and concentrations are tolerated. Only then should standard complex formulas be substituted, initially as small parts of the total feeding volume.

ASSOCIATED ANOMALIES

Nonfixation of the mesentery is the rule with this lesion, but a formal Ladd procedure[7] for malrotation is unnecessary, as the extensive postoperative adhesions will prevent mesenteric volvulus.

Atresias occasionally result from in utero ischemic necrosis. This results from strangulation of the mesenteric vessels by compression or angulation as they exit through the mural defect.

PROGNOSIS

Survival usually depends on prevention of or successful treatment for sepsis. When extensive bowel losses occur as the result of ischemic necrosis, survival may be difficult, but usually with prolonged TPN support adequate adaptation is possible.

DISCUSSION

Survival of this anomaly has increased remarkably in the last few years as a result of improved techniques of reconstruction, more vigorous volume restoration, better control of sepsis, and nutritional support with TPN.[98] Although successful treatment often requires a momentous effort, the resultant normal child is well worth it.

OMPHALOCELE

This entity differs from gastroschisis in that the intestine, although outside the abdomen, is contained within a peritoneal sac. It differs from gastroschisis in etiology[91] and in many aspects of management.

Omphalocele is a persistence of the normal herniation of the intestine into the extraembryonic coelom or, as is commonly stated, "into the cord." This occurs when, in early developmental stages, the gastrointestinal tract increases in length more rapidly than does the embryo, requiring it to loop outward from the as yet incompletely formed organism.[99]

Between 10 and 12 weeks of fetal life, with the fetus now more completely formed, the intestines normally return to the developed peritoneal cavity.[99] Failure to return, or incomplete or inaccurate return, results in persistence of herniation—the omphalocele. This may vary from the giant variety, which contains the entire intestine and more significantly the liver and is a major problem for surgical correction, to the tiny omphaloceles with minimal contained intestine. The latter are as easily repaired as an umbilical hernia.

A peritoneal sac is always present in omphalocele but may be ruptured during or after delivery. The cord structures come off the end of the sac, and the wall defect is directly at the umbilicus.

USUAL PRESENTATION

This baby presents with a midline defect in the exact umbilical area. Depending on the size of the defect, various amounts of the abdominal viscera are seen to be contained in a protruding peritoneal sac. This anomaly presents in essentially three forms: (a) a small to moderate defect containing only part of the intestine; (b) a large or giant defect containing most of the bowel, the liver, the spleen, and the pelvic organs (Fig 69); (c) a defect of any size, the peritoneal covering of which has been ruptured during or after delivery.

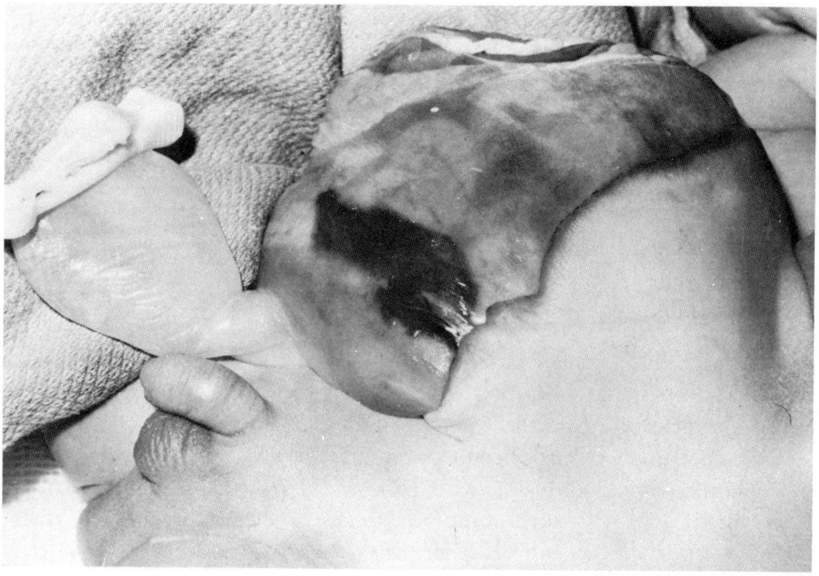

FIG. 69. A giant omphalocele containing bowel and liver. Note the umbilical cord coming from the sac that contains the abdominal contents.

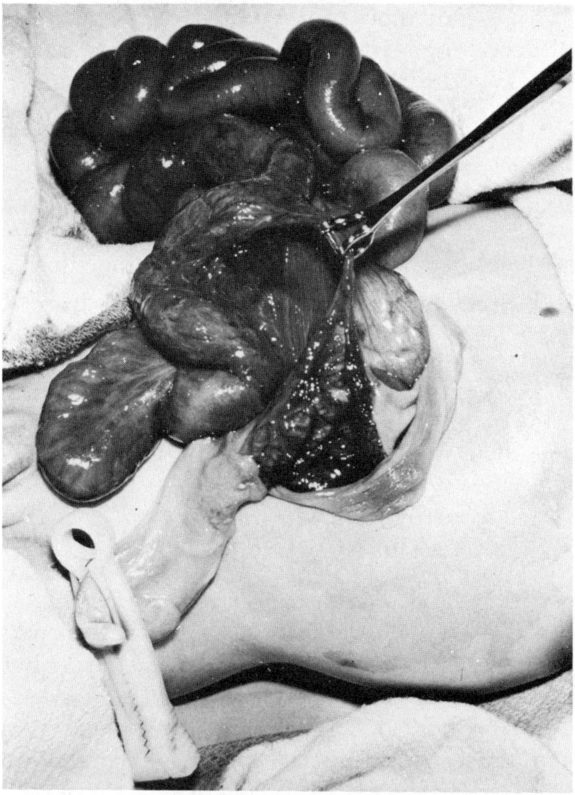

FIG. 70. A large, ruptured omphalocele. The membranes of the omphalocele sac are visible with the cord an extension of them. The bowel is not as thickened and adherent as is the bowel in gastroschisis (see Fig. 67).

DIAGNOSTIC TESTS

This lesion is easily recognized and requires no sophisticated diagnostic evaluation. Differentiation between ruptured omphalocele and gastrochisis may occasionally be difficult but is of no consequence in subsequent management (Fig. 70).

RESUSCITATION AND TRANSPORTATION REQUIREMENTS

The intact omphalocele presents none of the fluid and heat loss problems of gastroschisis. It needs only moist gauze protection and avoidance of trauma. The small omphalocele needs little more attention than an umbilical hernia. If the membrane is ruptured all the problems discussed under gastroschisis may apply.

PROPER HANDLING

Protection of the integrity of the sac should continue until a decision regarding the timing and method of repair is made. If the sac has ruptured, the baby should be treated in the same fashion, and with the same urgency, as he would if a gastroschisis were the problem.

Because omphalocele may be a manifestation of Beckwith-Weidemann syndrome,[100, 101] careful monitoring of blood sugar is important since the hypoglycemia common in this syndrome may be severe and prolonged.

CHOICE OF SURGICAL PROCEDURES

The choices here are more varied than with gastroschisis.

1. The skin may be closed over the intact peritoneal membrane. This results in a large ventral hernia requiring subsequent repair but usually will avoid sepsis in the high-risk newborn period.

2. Delayed initial repair can be achieved by drying and shrinking the sac. This is accomplished by painting the sac with Mercurochrome.[102] This technique is sometimes unsuccessful in reducing a giant omphalocele, and it may lead to an emergency repair in an infected wound if the sac degenerates.

3. Primary closure is preferred for all cases in which this is attainable. The limiting factor again is interference with respiration. Small and moderate-sized lesions can almost always be closed primarily. Stretching the abdominal wall will often facilitate this closure.

4. The giant omphalocele requires maximum effort and judgment to achieve closure. The problem is the extra-abdominal position of the liver. In these a combination of a poorly formed, inadequate-sized subdiaphragmatic space for containing the liver and an oversized globular organ makes reduction of the liver very difficult. Extreme stretching of the subcostal space and forceful reduction of the liver may be necessary. The risk of trauma to the liver with exsanguinating hemorrhage is high. However, if reduction of the liver is not achieved, it is subsequently all but impossible to return the herniated bowel to the peritoneal cavity. If reduction of the liver can be achieved, a prosthetic Silon* pouch will usually facilitate gradual reduction

*Silastic sheeting, Dow-Corning Corporation, Midland, Mich.

of the intestines over the next seven to ten days.[93-95] This avoids excessive respiratory embarrassment from pressure on the diaphragm (Fig. 71).

FACTORS OF IMPORTANCE IN POSTOPERATIVE CARE

When primary closure is achieved without excessive interference with respiratory function, postoperative care is uncomplicated. Routine attention to fluid management will suffice. Antibiotics are indicated as with all major procedures in infancy. When closure of a giant omphalocele is attempted, whether primarily or by staged reduction of a prosthetic pouch, major postoperative support of circulatory and respiratory dynamics will be required, including monitoring of arterial blood gases and central venous pressure. The discussion in the section on gastroschisis is fully applicable here.

ASSOCIATED ANOMALIES

Unlike gastroschisis, which is usually an isolated lesion, omphalocele may occur alone or may be either a part of a complex array of anomalies or one of

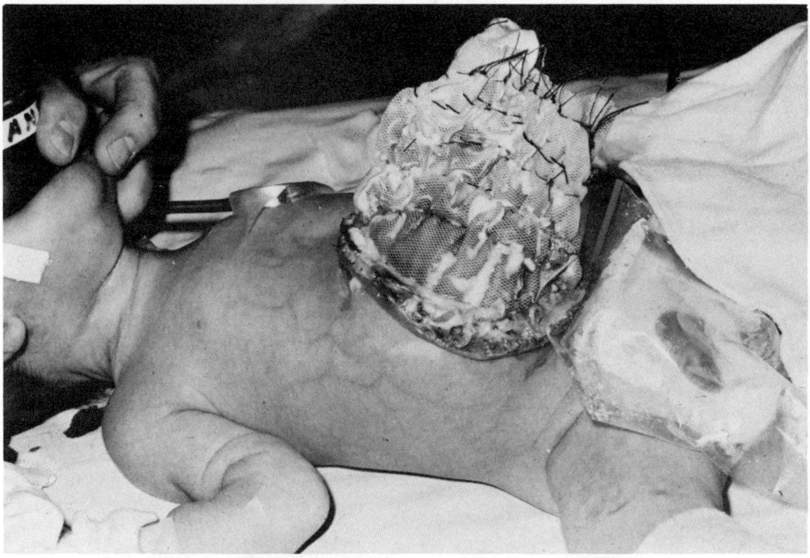

FIG. 71. Giant omphalocele in process of staged reduction using a synthetic pouch. Note the daily tightening of the pouch that has been accomplished, allowing gradual reduction of the viscera while allowing for respiratory adjustment.

numerous manifestations of a chromosomal defect such as Trisomy 13/15. It is frequently associated with exstrophy of the bladder and is a component of the Beckwith–Weidemann syndrome of visceral macrosomia and severe hypoglycemia.[100]

PROGNOSIS

Prognosis depends entirely on the ability to achieve proper closure without undue trauma to the liver and before sepsis can overwhelm the infant's resources. For the isolated omphalocele, once closure is achieved, long-term, problem-free survival is the rule. For the infant in whom omphalocele is only one manifestation of a complex chromosomal anomaly, survival depends on

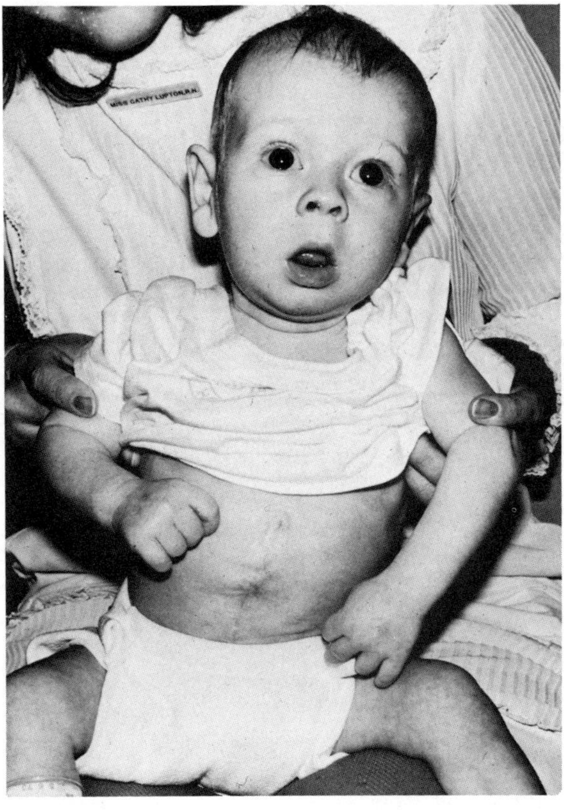

FIG. 72. Same infant as in Figure 71 after successful staged repair using a prosthetic pouch. Tracheostomy and ventilatory support were required during part of his course. The tracheostomy was removed when it was no longer required.

the other defects associated with the underlying chromosomal error. Many of these aberrations cause death early in infancy.

DISCUSSION

It has been difficult to evaluate treatment modalities for this lesion because most published series have either failed to differentiate between gastroschisis and omphalocele, have reported on omphaloceles of all sizes without regard to their unique problems and solutions, or have combined gastroschisis and all sizes of omphaloceles. Today, most gastroschisis patients and those with small to moderate-sized omphaloceles can be successfully managed with standard procedures and thoughtful pre- and postoperative care.

The giant omphalocele, with restricted peritoneal size and an eviscerated oversized globular liver, remains a striking challenge to the surgeon's skill, imagination, and intestinal fortitude (Fig. 72).

EXSTROPHY OF THE BLADDER

USUAL PRESENTATION

This entity is easily recognized (Fig. 73); no diagnostic maneuvers are necessary. The inexperienced physician is often confused by it and may misdiagnose it as a gastroschisis. The hypertrophied, irregularly folded bladder mucosa suggests bowel loops to him. Also, the associated epispadias leads to the impression of ambiguous genitalia. Improper sex identification may result.

DIAGNOSTIC TESTS

No diagnostic tests are needed initially. Eventually, x-ray studies of the sacrum and pelvis are needed to define associated skeletal abnormalities. Sacral defects, if present, portend possible neural deficits to the pelvic organs and lower extremities. Satisfactory evaluation of the urinary tract by intravenous pyelogram should be accomplished prior to discharge.

RESUSCITATION AND TRANSPORTATION REQUIREMENTS

The exposed bladder mucosa must be protected from drying. Vaseline gauze coverings usually suffice for this.

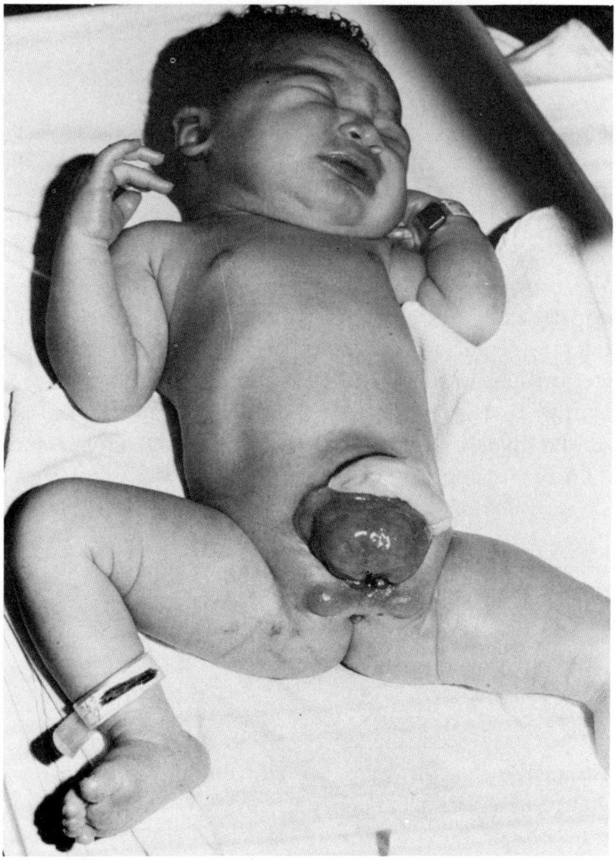

FIG. 73. Infant with exstrophy of the bladder.

PROPER HANDLING

The isolated exstrophy is not a serious management problem. Because the referring physician and the parents are usually upset by the appearance of the lesion, referral and transport are accomplished more expeditiously than for many life-threatening lesions that are hidden from view. Gracious acceptance and encouragement should be offered by the neonatal specialists.

CHOICE OF SURGICAL PROCEDURES

No surgical procedures are warranted in the immediate neonatal period. Eventually, a decision must be made for or against attempting to reconstruct the bladder. This is usually done between 6 and 18 months of life, but the recent trends are toward earlier surgery. Many surgeons have abandoned reconstructive efforts and prefer to remove the bladder and proceed to construction of a ureteroileal or ureterosigmoidal conduit.[103]

Although continence after reconstruction of the bladder is achieved infrequently, especially in males, these attempts at reconstruction usually are harmless as long as the upper urinary tracts are monitored and protected against the ravages of reflux, obstruction, and infection. The occasional success that avoids a lifelong urinary diversion is probably worth the efforts. Recently, with the use of a two-stage approach of initially repairing the bladder and subsequently the epispadias, results have been better in patients cared for by experienced teams.[104]

FACTORS OF IMPORTANCE IN POSTOPERATIVE CARE

Since this lies beyond the realm of immediate neonatal surgery, further discussion is not warranted here.

ASSOCIATED ANOMALIES

Exstrophy of the bladder can be associated with omphalocele alone or with the whole spectrum of complex multiple anomalies associated with chromosomal aberrations.

PROGNOSIS

Survival is to be expected for the patient with an isolated exstrophy. Complete surgical correction is infrequent but is more often successful in females.[104]

DISCUSSION

Complete correction of exstrophy requires a team effort by surgeons with expertise in neonatal urology, orthopedics, and pediatric surgery. It is best done by those with prior experience in the field. Too often, initial urinary diversions are performed by inexperienced general or urological surgeons. These ill-conceived procedures may make bladder reconstruction impossible and even satisfactory permanent diversions more difficult.

CYSTIC HYGROMA

USUAL PRESENTATION

The infant is born with a mass in the neck, usually in the posterior triangle. It is most often soft, cystic, and very large, sometimes extending anteriorly into the submandibular area as far as the trachea (Fig. 74).

DIAGNOSTIC TESTS

Chest roentgenograms should be obtained to search for evidence of mediastinal extension. Occasionally, a similar mass in the neck results from extension of a mediastinal thymic cyst.

Airway films (lateral x-rays of the neck) should be obtained to look for encroachment on the laryngeal or subglottic airspace. This is rare and does not occur with the large cysts of the typical cystic hygromas. Some of these lesions prove to be small-cyst-sized lymphangiomas, which "infiltrate" extensively among cervical tissues, and may involve the retropharyngeal area and the tissues of the larynx and airway.[105] Occasionally, the tongue is involved.[106]

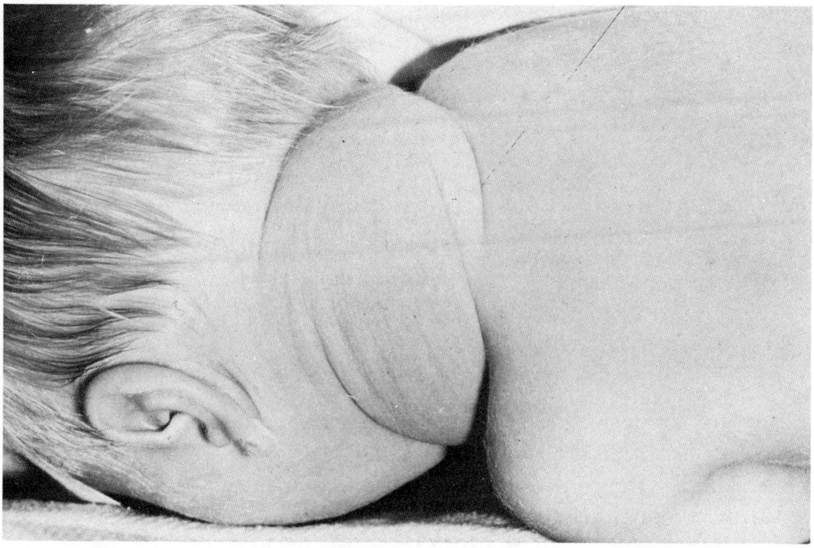

FIG. 74. Cystic hygroma of the cervical area in a newborn infant.

RESUSCITATION AND TRANSPORTATION REQUIREMENTS

Unless there is evidence of airway involvement, no special efforts or precautions are needed.

PROPER HANDLING

Because these lesions represent deformities of lymphatic vessels and communicate with the normal lymphatic clearing system, the incidence of infection is high. Antibiotic prophylaxis is indicated. Early surgical excision is preferable, once the baby is stable from any other neonatal complications. Airspace encroachment by an extensive pharyngeal lymphangioma must, of course, be treated appropriately with intubation if necessary. Eventually, tracheostomy may be required.

CHOICE OF SURGICAL PROCEDURES

Excision should be performed under general anesthesia with stable airway control through intubation. The typical hygromas with large cysts are usually easily removed and separated from surrounding tissues. Since this excision amounts essentially to a radical neck dissection in an infant, the surgeon must have precise knowledge of the anatomy of the region and experience in neck surgery if damage to important normal structures is to be avoided.

FACTORS OF IMPORTANCE IN POSTOPERATIVE CARE

Antibiotic coverage, usually with ampicillin, should be continued. We have found suction drainage to be very beneficial. It prevents accumulations of lymph and helps to hold the skin flaps in place. The potential for fluid accumulation and infection is great after this surgery because numerous lymphatic channels are divided without ligation. A most satisfactory suction drainage system can be fashioned by removing the proximal end from a butterfly needle–catheter set, cutting several holes in the tubing, and placing it as a suction catheter in the wound. Usually a single catheter beneath each skin flap suffices. If the butterfly needle is then inserted through the stopper of a vacuum blood-drawing tube,* a closed sterile suction system is achieved. The vacuum tubes are changed every 4 hours until drainage ceases (Fig. 75).

*Vacutainer, Becton, Dickinson & Co., Columbus, Neb.

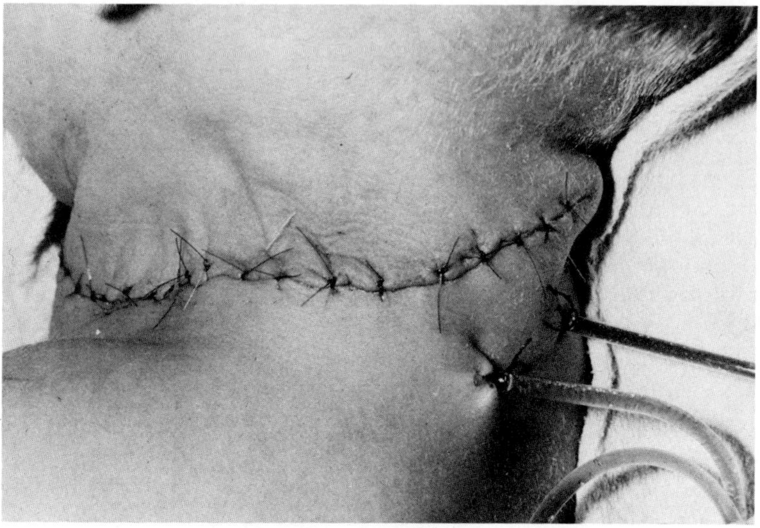

FIG. 75. Postoperative photograph of infant after excision of cystic hygroma. Suction drainage tubes are seen exiting through posterior stab wounds.

ASSOCIATED ANOMALIES

There are no anomalies associated with this entity.

PROGNOSIS

The large-cyst lesions can usually be removed completely. Recurrence is infrequent (Fig. 76). When the more extensively "infiltrating" small-cyst lymphangioma is found, total excision is difficult. This lesion represents extensive abnormality of the lymphatics of the tissues of a wide area. Complete excision is impossible because too much normal tissue is involved with the abnormal lymphatics. Recurrence (actually persistence) is more likely with these lesions. Infection is commonly the way the persistence is evidenced, but frequently the infection will help to scar and thereby reduce the amount of persistent tissue.

DISCUSSION

The fact that successful removal in the newborn period has been so frequent as to make it the preferred course needs reemphasis. Delay usually

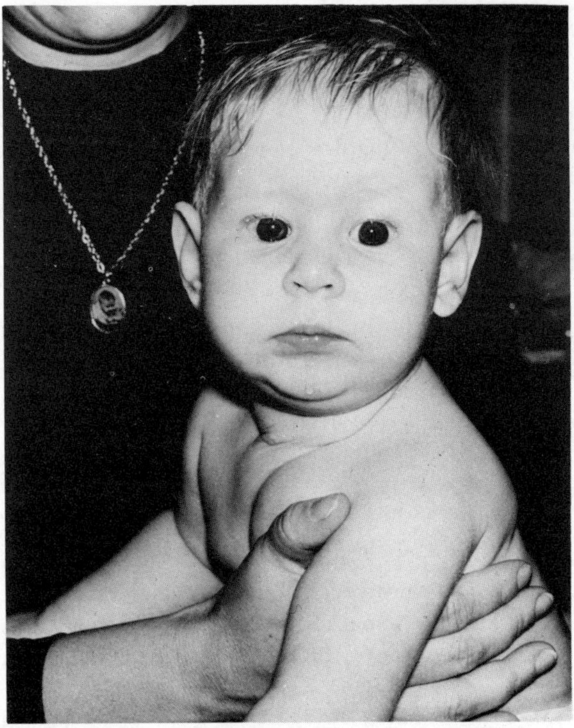

FIG. 76. Portrait of infant several months after excision of cystic hygroma. The cosmetic result is quite satisfactory.

leads to infection, which at best will make subsequent removal more difficult and more hazardous to the surrounding normal tissues.

SACROCOCCYGEAL TERATOMA

USUAL PRESENTATION

This is the most common tumor recognized immediately at birth. It is nevertheless rare, occurring in 1 in 40,000 births.[107] It may present as a midline mass arising from the sacrococcygeal region or be more to one side or the other and appear to arise in the gluteal tissue. Only part of the mass may be external, the remainder being intrapelvic. Occasionally, there is no external manifestation. The tumor arises from the anterior aspect of the coccyx, extending into the pelvis and up into the retroperitoneal abdomen (Fig. 77).

This tumor is usually irregular and variably cystic. It may be ruptured during or after delivery, in which case serious hemorrhage may result, requiring emergency excision. A history of twinning in the family is common. Females predominate, about 75 percent occurring in girls.[107,108]

DIAGNOSTIC TESTS

X-ray of the mass may show calcifications. Teeth or bones are occasionally noted. Films of the sacral spine will confirm its integrity and help to differentiate the teratoma from a meningomyelocele.

Other entities in the differential diagnosis include the following:

1. Buttock abscess, a most unlikely lesion with which to be born.
2. A lipoma of the cauda equina, which is usually associated with a capillary hemangioma in the sacral skin.
3. Other embryonal tumors that may arise within the pelvis such as rhabdomyosarcoma or neuroblastoma. Very rarely, these may extend out the sciatic notch into the buttock and present as buttock masses.

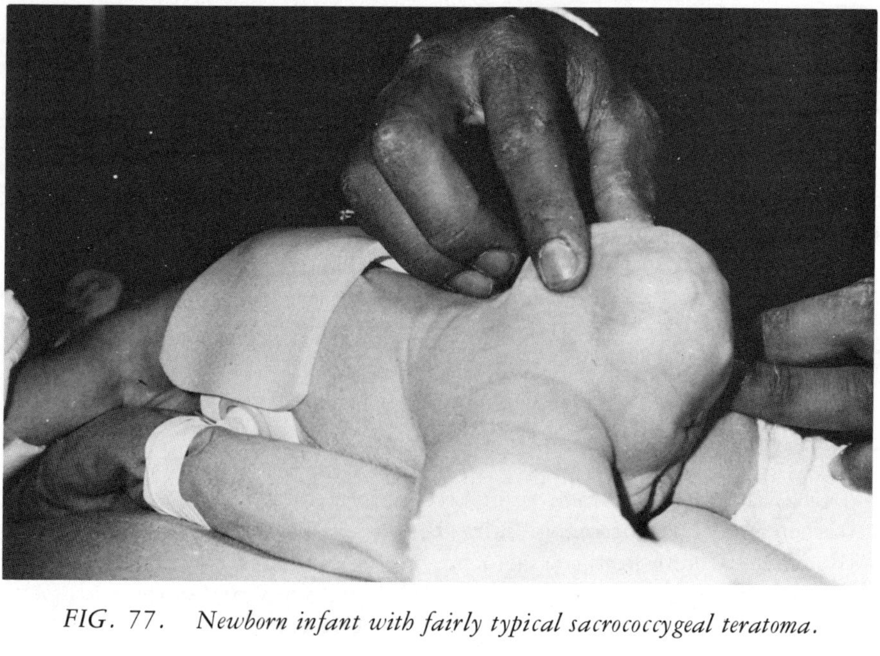

FIG. 77. Newborn infant with fairly typical sacrococcygeal teratoma.

The presence of the sacrococcygeal mass at birth makes teratoma the most likely diagnosis.

RESUSCITATION AND TRANSPORTATION REQUIREMENTS

Unless the skin is open and hemorrhage is a problem, simple protection from trauma and early transport are the only requirements.

PROPER HANDLING

Particularly when there is intrapelvic or intra-abdominal extension, an intravenous pyelogram should be performed. This will often show obstructive uropathy with dilated, tortuous ureters and hydronephrosis. Usually, these changes revert to normal within a few months after the obstruction is relieved.

Once the infant has stabilized from any attendant neonatal complications, operative removal is indicated. Delay gains nothing and may lead to complications such as rupture or hemorrhage. Long delay results in a high incidence of malignant degeneration. There is a fourfold increase in the incidence of malignancy[108] and a fivefold increase in mortality if excision is delayed beyond 1 month of life.[107] Beyond 2 months of age, one-half of the females and two-thirds of the males will have malignant tumors.[108]

CHOICE OF SURGICAL PROCEDURES

Wide, simple excision sparing all normal tissue but removing the coccyx is the indicated procedure. Failure to remove the coccyx leads to recurrence, and the recurrence may have malignant elements within it. A chevron-shaped incision placed between the coccyx and the anus gives excellent exposure and a most satisfactory cosmetic result. The rectum should be packed to aid in its subsequent identification. This will lessen the risk of injury to the rectum. Closure with suction catheters reduces the incidence of postoperative fluid collections and infection (see the subsection on factors of importance in postoperative care in the section on cystic hygroma).

FACTORS OF IMPORTANCE IN POSTOPERATIVE CARE

Attention to the wound to prevent fluid collections is the only requirement.

ASSOCIATED ANOMALIES

There are no specific associated anomalies, but there is an 18 percent incidence of associated congenital anomalies overall.[108]

PROGNOSIS

When excised in the newborn period in continuity with the coccyx, survival and functional results are excellent and recurrence rare. Malignant invasion and metastases are almost unheard of. After a few months' delay, however, malignant elements in the tumor tend to invade, and then the mortality is significant. From 5 to 15 percent of these teratomas are malignant when first seen.

There are few long-term problems with these patients. The cosmetic results are excellent. Some patients have occasional constipation, but, otherwise, complications or adverse sequelae are unusual (Fig. 78).

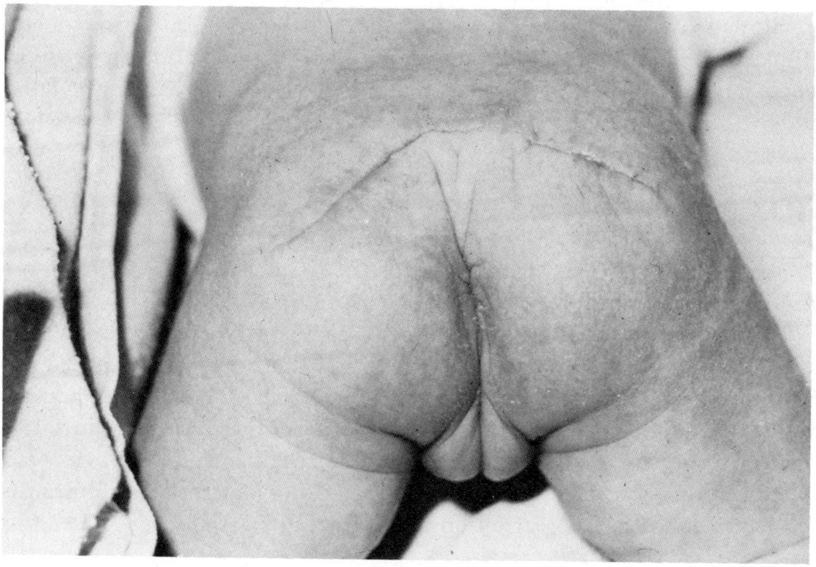

FIG. 78. Same infant as in Fig. 77 after excision of teratoma through a chevron-shaped incision. Suction drainage tubes as described in the section on cystic hygroma were used here as well.

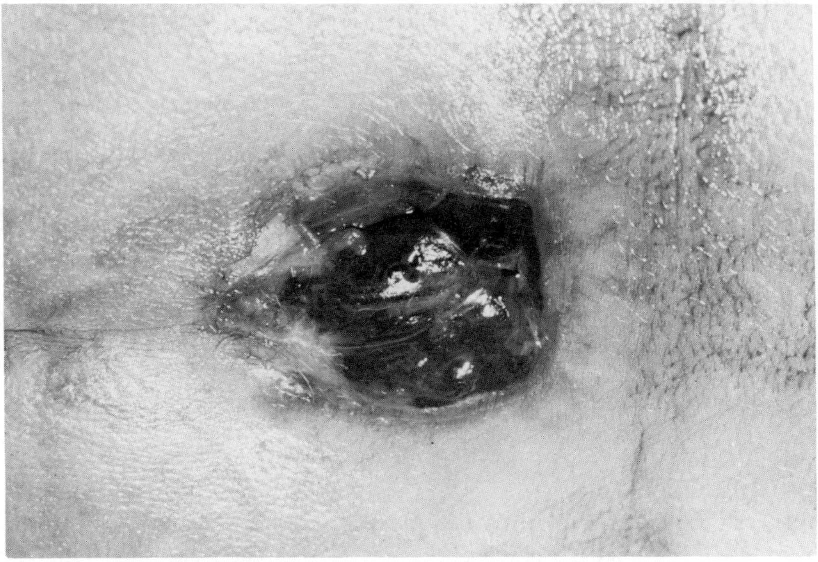

FIG. 79 Sacral meningomyelocele in a newborn infant.

MENINGOMYELOCELE/MENINGOCELE

This is one of the more common neurologic lesions of the newborn and is usually obvious at birth.

USUAL PRESENTATION

The baby is born with a variable-sized defect in the dorsum of the trunk. Meningocele is a defect of the soft tissues and bony vault with a protruding meningeal sac. The cord itself is intact. Usually there is no neurologic deficit. Meningomyelocele is a more serious anomaly involving the actual neural structures to various degrees.

These lesions may occur anywhere along the neural axis from the skull to the sacrum but are most common in the lower lumbar and sacral areas (Fig. 79).

DIAGNOSTIC TESTS

This lesion is obvious and initially requires no investigation. Subsequently, differentiation of meningocele from the more serious meningomyelocele is important.

RESUSCITATION AND TRANSPORTATION REQUIREMENTS

No resuscitation is usually required, but the lesion must be protected from drying, trauma, and contamination. Sterile, saline-soaked gauze covered with plastic wrap or vaseline gauze covered with sterile, dry gauze will suffice.

PROPER HANDLING

Inspection of the lesion often reveals the presence or absence of neural involvement. Continued coverage and protection is then desirable until early repair is accomplished. The major observation to be made is the level of neurologic functioning. When the anus is patulous and fails to "wink" in response to local painful stimuli and the lower extremities are flaccid or hypoactive, a major neurologic deficit is probably present. Some recovery may occur if any of the deficit is related to delivery contusion of the neural elements rather than to anomalous development.

Spinal radiographs should be obtained to evaluate the bony spine and the extent of defects in it. Baseline measurements of head circumference and evaluation of the fontanels for signs of increased intracranial pressure should be performed.

CHOICE OF SURGICAL PROCEDURES

As soon as the baby will tolerate anesthesia and surgery, closure of the defect in the neural coverings and the dorsal soft tissues should be accomplished. Local coverage may occasionally suffice, but usually a large rotation flap is needed to obliterate the defect. This procedure prevents dessication of the neural elements and avoids secondary deficits from trauma.

FACTORS OF IMPORTANCE IN POSTOPERATIVE CARE

The baby should be maintained in the prone position. Daily evaluation of the status of the wound is important to avoid fluid collections or unrecognized infection. Drainage should be afforded as needed.

ASSOCIATED ANOMALIES

Hydrocephalus is such a common accompanying problem as to be almost inseparable from the meningomyelocele.[109] Continuous reevaluation of head circumference and intracranial pressure is essential so that appropriate ventricular shunting procedures can be performed before brain damage occurs.

PROGNOSIS

Prognosis varies and depends primarily on the extent of neural deficit and the success of shunting procedures for hydrocephalus. Most patients with meningomyeloceles have considerable lower extremity, anorectal, and bladder innervation deficits, leaving them with lower extremity paresis and incontinence. However, most can lead productive lives and achieve reasonable physical status if cared for by a dedicated, well-organized myelodysplasia team of orthopedic, neurosurgical, urologic, and pediatric physicians and a host of paramedical personnel.

DISCUSSION

Some centers have been very aggressive with these children and have accomplished much with many of them. In other areas a more nihilistic view has predominated. The problem with nihilism is threefold:

1. Many of these children are mentally normal, and withholding treatment may destroy a mentally competent individual.

2. All untreated infants do not die, and some live for years as debilitated, incompetent individuals ravaged by hydrocephalus and deprived of the help they might have received.

3. Once we as physicians are willing to negotiate our commitment to saving each individual life, we open the door to untold numbers of considerations as to which lives are to be saved. Social ethics may then rapidly displace moral obligations.

ABDOMINAL AND FLANK MASSES

USUAL PRESENTATION

Abdominal and flank masses are usually found unexpectedly on physical examination. Even when they involve organs such as the kidney, which in older age groups may have associated signs and symptoms such as hematuria, these signs are almost never seen in newborn infants.[110]

Flank masses are usually relatively immobile. Intra-abdominal masses are highly mobile and often can be pushed from one quadrant to another.

DIAGNOSTIC TESTS

When the mass is a retroperitoneal one, intravenous pyelography will most often define its nature. Once an impression is gained from the pyelogram, additional studies can be planned. Table 1 in Section 2 is helpful in differentiating among the masses and suggesting definitive studies.

RESUSCITATION AND TRANSPORTATION REQUIREMENTS

No special procedures are usually needed.

CHOICE OF SURGICAL PROCEDURES

Malignant retroperitoneal masses and such benign lesions as duplications and mesenteric cysts should be excised once indicated diagnostic studies have been completed. The main preoperative consideration is to define those benign renal anomalies such as hydronephrosis which may not require surgery in the immediate newborn period.

FACTORS OF IMPORTANCE IN POSTOPERATIVE CARE

The specifics of these requirements will depend on the lesion involved. General postoperative support care is all that is usually required. Adjuvant chemotherapy and radiation will depend on the type and extent of the lesion and the surgical result. Most of the malignancies are being studied in national programs for determining useful adjuvant treatments.

ASSOCIATED ANOMALIES

No anomalies are associated with this lesion.

PROGNOSIS

Prognosis depends on the lesion, obviously, but particularly on whether it is malignant. Generally, however, even the most malignant lesions have an excellent prognosis in infancy. Great strides have been made, especially in Wilms' tumor.[111] Overall survival in this entity has been changed from 30 to over 80 percent for this malignancy in all age groups, and in infants prognosis for survival is almost 100 percent favorable.[112]

DISCUSSION

In past years, infants with abdominal masses have been rushed urgently to surgery. Today expeditious evaluation and planning are still indicated, but complete evaluation including baseline studies such as catecholamine levels should be obtained. Often arteriography will help to locate important vessels at the time of the operative procedure. Knowledge of the extent of involvement of major vessels may also help determine the timing and extent of operative procedures and sometimes dictate preoperative tumor reduction therapy by radiation or chemotherapy.[113]

Generally, the management of the lesions has been evolved by national study groups. Where combinations of treatment modalities have been successful, the exact modes of application of these techniques have been quite well defined. Where success has been less dramatic, carefully considered studies are in progress to obtain statistically valid data rapidly.

Each infant today should have the benefit of properly applied therapies by physicians experienced in the treatment of these lesions. This not only will ensure the best chance for cure, but also will allow application of recent knowledge of successful reduction of the needed doses of adjuvant modalities, most of which have some detrimental side effects along with their benefits.

Equally important, the opportunity to treat these patients within the context of national studies holds the best promise for future successes in those lesions not yet conquered. The national study groups involved in this work include the following:

1. Children's Cancer Study Group A
2. Acute Leukemia Group B

3. Southwest Oncology Group, Pediatric Division
4. National Wilms' Tumor Study

The studies that have been undertaken are as follows:

1. Wilms' tumor adjuvant therapies: all studies combined under group 4 above with other 3 groups participating
2. Neuroblastoma adjuvant therapy; mostly group 1 above
3. Rhabdomyosarcoma: intergroup studies (1, 2, and 3)
4. Hepatoblastoma: intergroup studies (1, 2, and 3)

CLEFT LIP AND PALATE

USUAL PRESENTATION

These lesions are obvious on physical examination. Either may occur independently or they may be combined. The extent of each varies from partial to complete clefts. When complete clefts of both the lip and palate occur, the cleft extends into the nares. Bilateral clefts occur.[114–116]

DIAGNOSTIC TESTS

No diagnostic tests are needed initially. Prior to treatment, definition of facial skeletal structure is important.

RESUSCITATION AND TRANSPORTATION REQUIREMENTS

Airway impairment is rarely a problem with these lesions. The Pierre Robin syndrome is an exception to this (see Section II). Otherwise, no special problems exist.

PROPER HANDLING

Early recognition and transport of these infants is usual. They are probably transported far more expeditiously than infants with many less obvious lesions that would benefit more from such rapidity. The infant should be stabilized and any neonatal complications attended to.

Most centers that frequently deal with these anomalies use a team approach to their care and have well-defined plans of treatment and preferred ages for repair. Usually, lips are repaired early in the infant's life, often during the initial hospitalization. Repair of the palate is usually delayed until later infancy, the exact age chosen for repair varying somewhat.[115,116]

CHOICE OF SURGICAL PROCEDURES

Usually, primary lip repair is performed. A prosthesis may be fashioned for temporary closure of the palatal defect. This aids feeding during early infancy until subsequent repair of the palate is performed.

FACTORS OF IMPORTANCE IN POSTOPERATIVE CARE

Protection of the lip after repair is important. Various splints and bars have been developed for this purpose, and each center has its favored program of postoperative wound protection and care. These should be diligently adhered to.

ASSOCIATED ANOMALIES

These may be isolated lesions, but they may also be part of complex multisystem or multiple midline anomalies. Some of these complex anomalies are chromosomally determined.

PROGNOSIS

Today generally excellent cosmetic results are being achieved. Complex palatal defects may be difficult to repair, and subsequently speech defects may require skilled attention from a team of specialists.

DISCUSSION

These lesions initially cause much concern to the parents and often to the primary physician as well. Therefore, early referral to a center experienced in their correction is warranted. The parents should be reassured regarding ultimate functional and cosmetic success, and a plan and time course of treatment should be outlined for them.

UMBILICAL ABNORMALITIES, URACHAL REMNANTS, AND OMPHALOMESENTERIC DUCT REMNANTS

Along with the umbilical vessels that provide interchange between the mother and fetus through the placenta, other structures traverse the umbilical area during development, and persistence of all or parts of these may result in anomalies with clinical significance. Most common among these are the omphalomesenteric or vitelline duct remnants, residua of the early embryonic yolk sac, and urachal remnants, parts of the urachal–allantoic stage of hindgut and cloacal formation.[117]

USUAL PRESENTATION

An omphalomesenteric remnant may persist as a wide open communication with the small bowel, in which case the umbilicus will have the appearance of a small "ostomy" with everted mucosa (Fig. 80). Alternatively, only a small sinus may persist, resulting in a persistent umbilical granuloma which may drain purulent or fecal-like material. Occult persistence of the omphalomesenteric duct may leave only a fibrous cord extending from a Meckel's diverticulum to the inner aspect of the umbilicus with no external manifestation. This cord may act as an axis for intestinal volvulus or may lead to mechanical obstruction if the bowel becomes entangled around it.

A persistent urachus may drain urine freely from the bladder, may simply drain purulent matter from a small sinus tract, or may present as a cyst-like structure between the bladder and the umbilicus. Abscess formation in the cystic remnant may be the initial presentation.

DIAGNOSTIC TESTS

Granulomas are common problems in the umbilicus. These represent failure of complete epithelialization of the wound left by the umbilical cord slough. Unusual appearing granulomas, mucosal-like areas, and fecal,

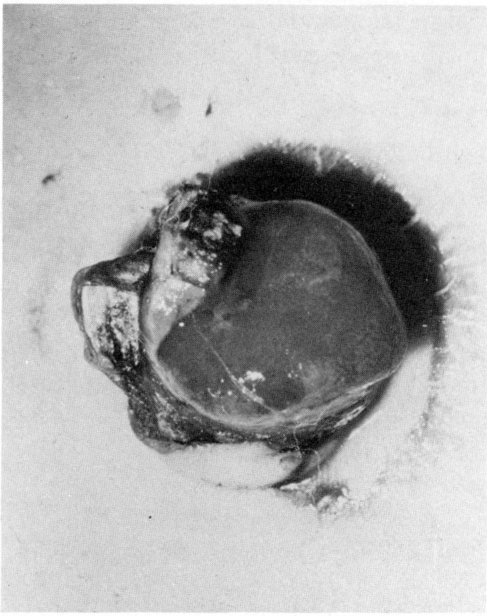

FIG. 80. Umbilical area of an infant with a persistent omphalomesenteric duct remnant. Note "ostomy-like" appearance.

urine-like, or copious purulent drainage should all lead to suspicion that anomalous remnants persist. If a sinus or actual enteric or urinary fistula is present, injection of a small amount of water-soluble medium will often demonstrate the lesion clearly on lateral abdominal radiographs. An intravenous pyelogram should be performed with suspicion or demonstration of a urachal anomaly. Superior "beaking" of the bladder on the pyelogram or on a cystogram will suggest that a urachal remnant is present. The tract itself may fill with dye if it is large enough. Gastrointestinal contrast radiographs will rarely show an omphalomesenteric remnant and are not worth the required radiation exposure.

RESUSCITATION AND TRANSPORTATION REQUIREMENTS

Special handling is rarely required. Often these babies are home before the diagnosis is suspected.

PROPER HANDLING

Infection, if present, must be treated appropriately. This may include initial incision and drainage of an infected urachal cyst. Otherwise, elective surgical correction is indicated.

CHOICE OF SURGICAL PROCEDURES

An omphalomesenteric remnant should be excised through a transverse infraumbilical incision. The remnant is freed from the umbilicus, dissected to the bowel, and removed completely, closing the intestinal defect transversely in layers. The umbilicus is reconstructed (Fig. 81).

Excision of a urachal tract or sinus can often be achieved through an infraumbilical incision with closure of the entry point into the bladder. Urachal cysts, especially when infected, may require a lower and larger incision for adequate exposure.

FACTORS OF IMPORTANCE IN POSTOPERATIVE CARE

Usual wound care and management of any resulting ileus or residual infection are the only requirements.

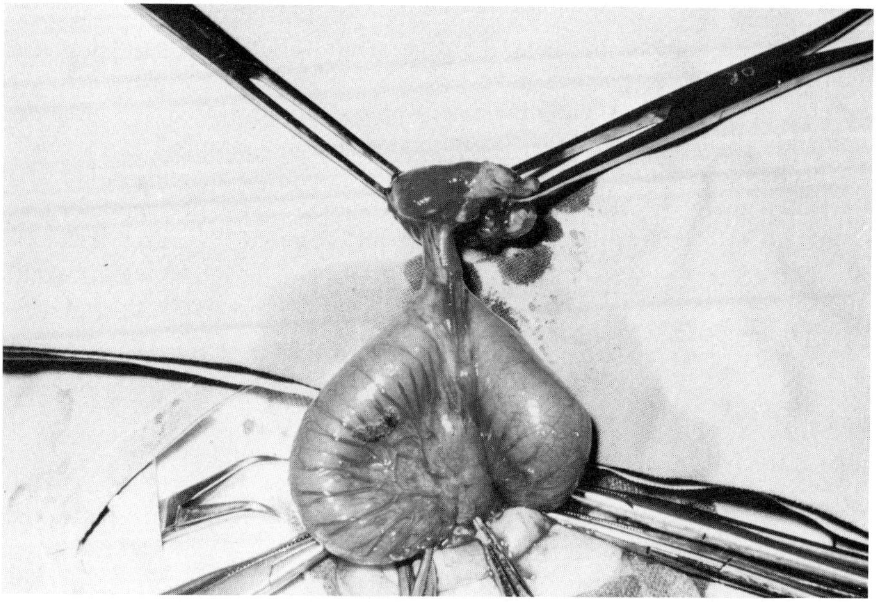

FIG. 81. Same infant as in Fig. 80 with remnant dissected to intestinal loop. Note the independent vascular supply from the mesentery.

ASSOCIATED ANOMALIES

No anomalies are associated with these lesions.

PROGNOSIS

Prognosis is excellent.

DISCUSSION

Although occasionally obvious, these lesions may be difficult to differentiate from an umbilical granuloma. Failure of a granuloma to resolve after one or two seemingly adequate cauterizations with silver nitrate should lead to further investigation for the presence of anomalous remnants.

The occult omphalomesenteric duct is actually a Meckel's diverticulum with a fibrous extention to the umbilicus. It may therefore present with any of the complications of the shorter diverticulum including hemorrhage, perforation, inflammation, and mechanical obstruction of the bowel. It is unlikely to act as the leading point of an intussusception, however.

INGUINAL HERNIA AND HYDROCELE

These lesions are common throughout childhood but are frequently seen in the neonatal nursery because the premature infant quite naturally has a persistently patent processus vaginalis testis.

USUAL PRESENTATION

An infant, often a premature infant, is noted to have a bulge in one or both inguinal areas or has a swollen scrotum, either unilaterally or bilaterally. These lesions may be obvious at birth or may become apparent at some subsequent time. The inguinal bulges may be present only with crying or straining or may be constantly apparent. The scrotal swelling may increase and decrease or remain constant. Occasionally, the first indication of the presence of a hernia in an infant is the incarceration of an intestinal loop.

DIAGNOSTIC TESTS

Physical examination and understanding of the developmental anatomy of the area are the most important factors in achieving proper diagnosis and treatment.

The differentiation of a hydrocele from a hernia in a child is a false one. Both represent persistent patency of the processus vaginalis testis beyond the usual late gestational obliteration of this entity. The frequency of these entities in premature infants is due to the fact that they are born before the processus normally obliterates. Once born, the normal intra-abdominal pressure relationships tend to keep the processus open.

If the opening from the general peritoneal cavity into its finger-like inguinal extension is narrow, only fluid can pass from the main peritoneal cavity to the inguinal and scrotal region, so that a "hydrocele" results. When the opening is very narrow over a long segment, fluid will not return readily to the peritoneal cavity, creating an enlarging balloon-like scrotal "hydrocele."

Larger tracts will allow slow resolution of the fluid so that the hydrocele changes size. When the opening is quite wide, large amounts of fluid can enter and return instantaneously, demonstrating a clear-cut hernia. Loops of bowel may readily enter as well. In a female infant the tube or ovary may enter the hernia sac and may easily become incarcerated.

Hernias and hydroceles must be differentiated from undescended testicle, torsion of a testicle, and testicular tumors. The latter are very rare, especially in the neonatal period.[118] A fully open hernia is easily identified by its ease of reduction. An incarcerated hernia can be confirmed by the thickened mass running all the way up to the internal ring, by lack of transillumination, and frequently by palpating at rectal examination, a loop of bowel entering the inguinal ring. Radiographs of the inguinal area may show gas in the inguinal canal or scrotum, confirming the presence of incarcerated bowel. A hydrocele has a rounded upper aspect and does not extend into the internal ring. It clearly transilluminates. An undescended testicle can be suspected when no testicle can be identified in the scrotum. A hernia is an almost universally associated anomaly with an undescended testicle,[119] but the hernia is rarely clinically apparent in the newborn period.

RESUSCITATION AND TRANSPORTATION REQUIREMENTS

Unless the hernia contains incarcerated intestine, no resuscitation is needed. The severity of incarceration is variable, and reduction of the more tightly incarcerated loops requires more experienced surgeons. Almost all can be reduced if properly evaluated and manipulated. Reduction is preferable to operating on an incarcerated hernia in a small infant, as that procedure is fraught with hazards and complications.[120]

PROPER HANDLING

If an unincarcerated hernia is present, it should be repaired whenever the baby will tolerate surgery and anesthesia. Waiting months for the baby to grow up only risks incarceration and more serious problems related to injury to the bowel or testicle.

If a hydrocele is present at birth and does not change in size, observation for six months is indicated. In this instance the processus may have filled with fluid and then the opening may have closed. The fluid-filled sac may gradually subside and obliterate. Persistence beyond six months, emptying and refilling, or gradual enlargement indicate persistent patency to the main peritoneal cavity.[121] Herniorrhaphy is then indicated.

A hydrocele developing after birth must have a patent processus connecting to the main peritoneal cavity. The indications for surgery are as follows:

1. The risk of bowel incarceration if the upper part of the processus is widely patent with the narrowing in the midportion

2. The frequency of gradual persistent enlargement and distortion of scrotal tissues making subsequent repair and resolution more difficult

3. The possibility of hemorrhage into the hydrocele from stretching and rupturing an adjacent vessel

CHOICE OF SURGICAL PROCEDURES

Repair of a child's hernia or hydrocele should be a short, simple procedure utilizing a small skin crease incision, a minimal, atraumatic dissection of normal tissues, a thorough identification of the hernia sac, complete separation of it back to the internal ring, and a high ligation and excision of the sac. Careful closure with attention to cosmetically important details should complete the operation. A repair of the direct wall is rarely indicated unless the surgeon has damaged the otherwise healthy intact tissues.[121]

The question of "blind" exploration of a clinically normal opposite side must be individualized and based on the patient's condition generally and during surgery, the surgeon's skill and experience, and the desires of the parents after reasonably informed discussion. Hard and fast rules here are inappropriate and potentially dangerous.

FACTORS OF IMPORTANCE IN POSTOPERATIVE CARE

Properly done, the procedure requires nothing but moderate protection of the wound until it heals. We use a subcuticular absorbable suture and a collodion dressing, which prevents soilage.

ASSOCIATED ANOMALIES

This lesion is so common that it may be associated with any other anomaly, but none are consistently associated with it.

PROGNOSIS

Recurrences should be negligible and the complication rate miniscule.

DISCUSSION

The danger of necrosis of the bowel from incarceration in a hernia sac, although real, has been much overemphasized relative to the almost total deemphasis of the more significant risk of occlusion of the testicular blood supply and ischemic necrosis and atrophy of the testicle.[122] The tiny vascular supply to the testicle is easily occluded when bowel becomes incarcerated in the internal ring. The bowel is better protected by its thick wall and extensive anastomotic blood supply. Occasionally, even when the incarcerated bowel is relatively easily reduced, the testicle may go on to atrophy.

Millions of babies have been safely managed through anesthesia and surgery in experienced hands with a very low rate of complications. Nonetheless, herniorrhaphy in an infant remains a difficult and potentially damaging procedure, frequently taxing the skill of the most experienced pediatric surgeon. It should not be undertaken by untrained and inexperienced surgeons just because hernias are common. Every child's hernia cannot be taken care of in a major center by a pediatric surgeon, but perhaps those in prematures and small infants should be. For bigger, older infants, thousands of general surgeons have been taught, during residency rotations on pediatric surgical services, to perform infant herniorrhaphies properly and safely. It is to them that communities without a pediatric surgeon should look for safe management of infant hernias.

UNDESCENDED TESTICLE

This is a frequent finding in premature infants, and questions arise as to proper management.

USUAL PRESENTATION

The baby, especially a premature infant, may have one or both testicles absent from the scrotum.

DIAGNOSTIC TESTS

First an attempt should be made to locate the testicle. If it can be manipulated into the scrotum, it is a *retractile* rather than an undescended testicle. In older infants and children, sitting them up with the soles of their feet together and knees widely abducted will release the cremasteric reflex and allow the retractile testicles to descend into the scrotum. Most of these children will have retractile, not cryptorchid, testicles.

RESUSCITATION AND TRANSPORTATION REQUIREMENTS

There are no requirements.

PROPER HANDLING

Premature infants frequently have undescended testicles. Nothing need be done during the first year of life unless a clinically apparent hernia is present. Most of these testicles in premature infants will descend subsequently during the first months of life. If a testicle fails to descend by the age of 2 years, surgery should be planned shortly thereafter.

DISCUSSION

Although a common finding in the high-risk nursery, undescended testicles require no treatment in the newborn period. However, an accompanying hernia should be repaired, and, as part of that procedure, orchidopexy should be performed.

When the hernia is not clinically apparent, waiting until the child is 2 years of age is appropriate. After that time, descent is unlikely and the incidence of fibrotic degeneration of the spermatogonia increases yearly.[123]

Hormone injections and "waiting until puberty" will not achieve descent of a truly undescended testicle, because it is anatomically impossible for it to descend.[124]

REFERENCES

1. Mustard WT, Ravitch MM, Snyder WH, Jr, et al: Pediatric Surgery. Chicago, Year Book, 1969
2. Swenson O (ed): Pediatric Surgery, 3rd ed. New York, Appleton, 1969
3. Gans SL (ed): Surgical Pediatrics. New York, Grune and Stratton, 1973
4. Baran EM, Houston HE, Lynn HB, et al: Foramen of Morgagni hernias in children. Surgery 62:1076, 1967
5. Johnson DG, Deaner RM, Koop CE: Diaphragmatic hernia in infancy: factors affecting the mortality rate. Surgery 62:1082, 1967
6. Snyder WH, Jr, Greaney EM: Congenital diaphragmatic hernia: 77 consecutive cases. Surgery 57:576, 1965
7. Ladd WE, Gross RE: Abdominal Surgery of Infancy and Childhood. Philadelphia, Saunders, 1941, p 62
8. Padula RT: Postoperative management. In Sabiston DC, Jr, Spencer FC (eds): Gibbon's Surgery of the Chest. Philadelphia, Saunders, 1976, p 176
9. Holder TM, Cloud DT, Lewis JE, Jr, et al: Esophageal atresia and tracheoesophageal fistula: a survey of its members by the Surgical Section of the American Academy of Pediatrics. Pediatrics 34:542, 1964
10. Koop CE, Hamilton JP: Atresia of the esophagus: factors affecting survival in 249 cases. Z Kinderchir 5:319, 1968
11. Ty TC, Brunet C, Beardmore HE: A variation in the operative technic for the treatment of esophageal atresia with tracheosophageal fistula. J Pediatr Surg 2:118, 1967
12. Touloukian RJ, Pickett LK, Spackman T, et al: Repair of esophageal atresia by end-to-side anastomosis and ligation of the tracheoesophageal fistula: a critical review of 18 cases. J Pediatr Surg 9:305, 1974
13. Ein SH, Theman TE: A comparison of the results of primary repair of esophageal atresia with tracheoesophageal fistulas using end-to-side and end-to-end anastomosis. J Pediatr Surg 8:641, 1973
14. Abrahamson J, Shandling B: Esophageal atresia in the underweight baby: a challenge. J Pediatr Surg 7:608, 1972
15. Ashcraft KW, Goodwin C, Amoury RA, et al: Early recognition and aggressive treatment of gastroesophageal reflux following repair of esophageal atresia. J Pediatr Surg 12:317, 1977
16. Azar H. Chrispin AR, Waterston DJ: Esophageal replacement with transverse colon in infants and children. J Pediatr Surg 6:3, 1971
17. Waterston DJ: Reconstruction of the esophagus. In Mustard WT, Ravitch MM, Snyder WH, Jr, et al (eds): Pediatric Surgery. Chicago, Year Book, 1969, p 400
18. Ein SH, Shandling B, Simpson JS, et al: A further look at the gastric tube as an esophageal replacement in infants and children. J Pediatr Surg 8:859, 1973
19. Heimlich HJ: Esophageal replacement with a reversed gastric tube. Dis Chest 36:478, 1959
20. Hendren WH, Hale JR: Esophageal atresia treated by electromagnetic bougienage and subsequent repair. J Pediatr Surg 11:713, 1976

21. Gans SL, Berci G: Inside tracheoesophageal fistula: new endoscopic approaches. J Pediatr Surg 8:205, 1973

22. Bedard P, Girvan DP, Shandling B: Congenital H-type tracheosophageal fistula. J Pediatr Surg 9:663, 1974

23. Novoselac M, Dangel P, Fisch U: Laryngotracheoesophageal cleft. J Pediatr Surg 8:963, 1973

24. Pettersson G: Inhibited separation of larynx and the upper part of trachea from oesophagus in a newborn. Acta Chir Scand 110:250, 1955

25. Burroughs N, Leape LL: Laryngotracheoesophageal cleft: report of a case successfully treated and review of the literature. Pediatrics 53:516, 1974

26. Javett SL, Jackson H, Utian HL: Torgersen's muscle and infantile hypertrophic pyloric stenosis. J Pediatr Surg 8:383, 1973

27. Simpson AJ, Leonidas JC, Krasna IH, et al: Roentgen diagnosis of midgut malrotation. Value of upper gastrointestinal radiographic study. J Pediatr Surg 7:243, 1972

28. Berdon WE, Baker DH, Bull S, et al: Midgut malrotation and volvulus: which films are most helpful. Radiology 96:375, 1970

29. Lynn HB: Duodenal obstruction: atresia, stenosis and annular pancreas. In Mustard WT, Ravitch MM, Snyder WH Jr, et al (eds): Pediatric Surgery. Chicago, Year Book, 1969, p 800

30. Feuchtwanger MM, Weiss Y: Side-to-side duodenoduodenostomy for obstructing annular pancreas in the newborn. J Pediatr Surg 3:398, 1968

31. Bishop HC, Filston HC: An inversion-ligation technique for incidental appendectomy. J Pediatr Surg 8:889, 1973

32. Lilly JR, Randolph JG: Total inversion of the appendix: experiences with incidental appendectomy in children. J Pediatr Surg 3:357, 1968

33. Aitken J: Congenital intrinsic duodenal obstruction in infancy. A series of 30 cases treated over a 6 year period. J Pediatr Surg 1:546, 1966

34. Bodian M, White LLR, Carter CO, et al: Congenital duodenal obstruction and mongolism. Br Med J 1:77, 1952

35. Louw JH, Barnard CN: Congenital intestinal atresia: observations on its origin. Lancet 2:1065, 1955

36. Louw JH: Resection and end-to-end anastomosis in the management of atresia and stenosis of the small bowel. Surgery 62:940, 1967

37. Filston HC, Johnson DG: Percutaneous venous cannulation in neonates and infants: a method for catheter insertion without "cut-down." Pediatrics 48:896, 1971

38. Benson CD, Lloyd JR, Krabbenhoff KL: The surgical and metabolic aspects of massive small bowel resection in the newborn. J Pediatr Surg 2:227, 1967

39. Howat JM, Aaronson I: Sugar intolerance in neonatal surgery. J Pediatr Surg 6:719, 1971

40. Santulli TV: Meconium ileus. In Mustard WT, Ravitch MM, Snyder WH, Jr, et al (eds): Pediatric Surgery. Chicago, Year Book, 1969, p 851

41. Martin DJ: Experiences with acute surgical conditions. Radiol Clin North Am 13:297, 1975

42. Noblett HR: Treatment of uncomplicated meconium ileus by Gastrografin enema: a preliminary report. J Pediatr Surg 4:190, 1969

43. Wagget J, Bishop HC, Koop CE: Experience with Gastrografin enema in the treatment of meconium ileus. J Pediatr Surg 5:649, 1970

44. Rowe MI, Seagram G, Weinberger M: Gastrografin induced hypertonicity: the pathogenesis of a neonatal hazard. Am J Surg 125:185, 1973

45. Leonidas JC, Burry VF, Fellows RA: Possible adverse effect of methyl glucamine diatrizoate compounds on the bowel of newborn infants with meconium ileus. Radiology 121:693, 1976

46. Lutzger LG, Factor SM: Effects of some water-soluble contrast media on the colonic mucosa. Radiology 118:545, 1976

47. Bishop HC, Koop CE: Management of meconium ileus: resection, Roux-en-Y anastomosis and ileostomy irrigation with pancreatic enzymes. Ann Surg 145:410, 1957

48. Meeker IA, Jr, Kincannon WN: Acetylcysteine used to liquify inspissated meconium causing intestinal obstruction in the newborn. Surg 56:419, 1964

49. Cordonnier JK, Izant RJ, RJ, Jr: Meconium ileus equivalent. Surgery 54:667, 1963

50. Matthews LW, Doershuk CF, Wise M, et al: A therapeutic regimen for patients with cystic fibrosis. J Pediatr 65:558, 1964

51. diSant'Agnese PA, Blanc WA: Distinctive type of biliary cirrhosis of liver associated with cystic fibrosis of the pancreas: recognition through signs of portal hypertension. Pediatrics 18:387, 1956

52. Stern RC, Stevens DP, Boat TF, et al: Symptomatic hepatic disease in cystic fibrosis: incidence, course, and outcome of portal systemic shunting. Gastroenterology 70:645, 1976

53. Yoo RP, Touloukian RJ: Intussusception in the newborn: a unique clinical entity. J Pediatr Surg 9:495, 1974

54. Ravitch MM: Intussusception. In Mustard WT, Ravitch MM, Snyder WH, Jr, et al (eds): Pediatric Surgery. Chicago, Year Book, 1969, p 914

55. Bailey RJ, Jr, Burgert EO, Jr, Dahlin DC: Malignant lymphoma in children. Pediatrics 28:985, 1961

56. Blackburn WW, Filston HC: Common symptoms in children: routine illness or abdominal lymphoma. Am J Surg 130:539, 1975

57. Grosfeld JL, Berman IR: Toxic factors in experimental ileo-ileal intussusception. Presented before the 4th Annual Meeting of the American Pediatric Surgical Society, Phoenix, April 1973.

58. Raflo GT, Jones RCW, Jr, Wangensteen SL: Inadequacy of steriods in treatment of severe hemorrhagic shock. Am J Surg 130:321, 1975

59. Ein SH: Recurrent intussusception in children. J Pediatr Surg 10:751, 1975

60. Swenson O, Sherman JO, Fisher JH: Diagnosis of congenital megacolon: an analysis of 501 patients. J Pediatr Surg 8:587, 1973

61. Poole CA, Rowe MI: Distal neonatal intestinal obstruction: the choice of contrast material. J Pediatr Surg 11:1011, 1976

62. Davis WS, Campbell JB: Neonatal small left colon syndrome. Am J Dis Child 129:1024, 1975

63. Philippart AI, Reed JO, Georgeson KE: Neonatal small left colon syndrome. J Pediatr Surg 10:733, 1975

64. Hope JW, Borns PF, Berg PK: Roentgenologic manifestations of Hirschsprung's disease in infancy. Am J Roentgenol Radium Ther Nucl Med 95:217, 1965

65. Pilling GP, Cresson SL: Hirschsprung's disease. In Mustard WT, Ravitch MM, Snyder WH, Jr, et al (eds): Pediatric Surgery. Chicago, Year Book, 1969, p 967

66. Swenson O, Bill AH, Jr: Resection of rectum and rectosigmoid with preservation of the sphincter for benign spastic lesions producing megacolon. Surgery 24:212, 1948

67. Duhamel B: A new operation for the treatment of Hirschsprung's disease. AMA Arch Dis Child 35:38, 1960

68. Martin LW, Caudill DR: A method for elimination of the blind rectal pouch in the Duhamel operation for Hirschsprung's disease. Surgery 62:951, 1967

69. Soper RT, Figueroa PR: Surgical treatment of Hirschsprung's disease: comparison of modifications of the Duhamel and Soave operations. J Pediatr Surg 6:761, 1971

70. Soave F: Hirschsprung's disease: a new surgical technique. AMA Arch Dis Child 39:116, 1964

71. Boley S: New modification of the surgical treatment of Hirschsprung's disease. Surgery 56:1015, 1964

72. Boley S: An endorectal pullthrough operation with primary anastomosis for Hirschsprung's disease. Surg Gynecol Obstet 127:353, 1968

73. Swenson O, MacMahon HE, Jagues WE, et al: New concept of etiology of magaloureters. N Engl J Med 246:41, 1952

74. Clatworthy HW, Howard WHR, Lloyd J: The meconium plug syndrome. Surgery 39:131, 1956

75. Ellis DG, Clatworthy HW: The meconium plug syndrome-revisited. J Pediatr Surg 1:54, 1966

76. Kock NG, Darle N, Dotevall G: Inhibition of intestinal motility in man by glucagon given intraportally. Gastroenterology 53:88, 1967

77. Wangensteen DA, Rice CO: Imperforate anus: a method of determining the surgical approach. Ann Surg 92:77, 1930

78. Stephens FD, Smith ED: Ano-Rectal Malformations in Children. Chicago, Year Book, 1971

79. Miller RC: The perineal pearl—a sign in imperforate anus. Presented before the 5th Annual Meeting, American Pediatric Surgical Association, New Orleans. Apr 5, 19/4

80. Santulli TV, Kiesewetter WB, Bill AH, Jr: Anorectal anomalies: a suggested international classification. J Pediatr Surg 5:281, 1970

81. Ramenofsky ML, Raffensperger JG: An abdomino-perineal-vaginal pullthrough for definitive treatment of hydrometrocolpos. J Pediatr Surg 6:381, 1971

82. Boix-Oschoa J: Meconium peritonitis. J Pediatr Surg 3:715, 1968

83. Gross S, Melhorn D: Exchange transfusion with citrated whole blood for disseminated intravascular coagulation. J Pediatr 78:415, 1971

84. Miller RE: Perforated viscus. A new radiological sign. Radiology 74:65, 1960

85. Bell MJ, Kosloske AM, Benton C, et al: Neonatal necrotizing enterocolitis: prevention of perforation. J Pediatr Surg 8:601, 1973

86. Dudgeon DL, Coran AG, Lauppe FA, et al: Surgical management of acute necrotizing enterocolitis in infancy. J Pediatr Surg 8:607, 1973

87. Touloukian RJ, Berdon WE, Amoury RA, et al: Surgical experience with necrotizing enterocolitis in the infant. J Pediatr Surg 2:389, 1967

88. Krasna IH, Becker JM, Schneider KM, et al: Colonic stenosis following necrotizing enterocolitis of the newborn. J Pediatr Surg 5:200, 1970

89. Lloyd DA, Cywes S: Intestinal stenosis and enterocyst formation as late complications of neonatal necrotizing enterocolitis. J Pediatr Surg 8:479, 1973

90. Stein H, Kavin I, Faerber EN: Colonic strictures following nonoperative management of necrotizing enterocolitis. J Pediatr Surg 10:943, 1975

91. Izant RJ, Jr, Brown F, Rothmann BF: Current embryology and treatment of gastroschisis and omphalocele. Arch Surg 93:49, 1966

92. Raffensperger JG, Jona JZ: Gastroschisis. Surg Gynecol Obstet 138:230, 1974

93. Schuster SR: A new method for the staged repair of large omphaloceles. Surg Gynecol Obstet 125:837, 1967

94. Allen RG, Wrenn EL, Jr: Silon as a sac in the treatment of omphalocele and gastroschisis. J Pediatr Surg 4:3, 1969

95. Hollabaugh RS, Boles ET, Jr: The management of gastroschisis. J Pediatr Surg 8:263, 1973

96. Filston HC, Izant RJ, Jr: Translocation of the umbilical artery to the lower abdomen: an adjunct to the postoperative monitoring of arterial blood gases in major abdominal wall defects. J Pediatr Surg 10:225, 1975

97. Morgan WW, Jr, Harkins GA: Percutaneous introduction of long-term indwelling venous catheters in infants. J Pediatr Surg 7:538, 1972

98. Filler RM, Eraklis AJ, Das JB, et al: Total intravenous nutrition (an adjunct to the management of infants with a ruptured omphalocele). Am J Surg 121:454, 1971

99. Moore KL: The Developing Human. Clinically Oriented Embryology. Philadelphia, Saunders, 1973, p 183

100. Beckwith JB: Extreme cytomegaly of the adrenal fetal cortex, omphalocele, hyperplasia of kidneys and pancreas, and Leydig-cell hyperplasia—another syndrome? Presented at the Annual Meeting of Western Society for Pediatric Research, Los Angeles, Nov 11, 1963.

101. Sotela-Avila C. Singer DB: Syndrome of hyperplastic fetal visceromegaly and neonatal hypoglycemia (Beckwith syndrome). Pediatrics 46:240, 1970

102. Grob M: Conservative treatment of exomphalos. AMA Arch Dis Child 38:148, 1963

103. Hays DM: Urinary diversion. In Mustard WT, Ravitch MM, Snyder WH, Jr, et al (eds): Pediatric Surgery. Chicago, Year Book, 1969, p 1238

104. Chisolm TC: Exstrophy of the urinary bladder. In Mustard WT, Ravitch MM, Snyder WH, Jr, et al (eds): Pediatric Surgery. Chicago, Year Book, 1969, p 1213

105. Harkins GA, Sabiston DC, Jr: Lymphangioma in infancy and childhood. Surgery 47:811, 1960

106. Koop CE, Moschakis EA: Capillary lymphangioma of the tongue complicated by glossitis. Pediatrics 27:800, 1961

107. Izant RJ, Jr, Filston HC: Sacrococcygeal teratoma. Analysis of forty-three cases. Am J Surg 130:617, 1975

108. Altman RP, Randolph JG, Lilly JR: Sacrococcygeal teratoma. American Academy of Pediatrics Surgical Section Survey, 1973. J Pediatr Surg 9:389, 1974

109. McQueen JD: Congenital anomalies of the neuraxis and related maldevelopment disorders. In Mustard WT, Ravitch MM, Snyder WH, Jr (eds): Pediatric Surgery. Chicago, Year Book, 1969, p 1514

110. Snyder WH, Jr., Hastings TN, Pollock WF: Retroperitoneal tumors. In Mustard WT, Ravitch MM, Snyder WH, Jr, et al (eds): Pediatric Surgery. Chicago, Year Book, 1969, p 1020

111. Johnson DG, Maceira DG, Koop CE: Wilms' tumor treated with actinomycin D: the relationship of age and extent of disease to survival. J Pediatr Surg 2:13, 1967

112. D'Angio GT, Evans AE, Breslow N, et al: The treatment of Wilms' tumor: results of the national Wilms' tumor study. Cancer 38:633, 1976

113. Wagget J, Koop CE: Wilms' tumor: preoperative radiotherapy and chemotherapy in the management of massive tumors. Cancer 26:338, 1970
114. Matthews DN: Hare lip and cleft palate. In Mustarde JC (ed): Plastic Surgery in Infancy and Childhood. Philadelphia, Saunders, 1971 p 1
115. Fryer MP, Brown JB: Cleft lip. In Mustard WT, Ravitch MM, Snyder WH, Jr, et al (eds): Pediatric Surgery. Chicago, Year Book, 1969, p 162
116. Lindsay WK: Cleft palate. In Mustard WT, Ravitch MM, Snyder WH, Jr, et al (eds): Pediatric Surgery. Chicago, Year Book, 1969, p 170
117. Moore KL: The Developing Human. Clinically Oriented Embryology. Philadelphia, Saunders, 1973, p 204
118. Houser R, Izant RJ, Jr, Persky L: Testicular tumors in children. Am J Surg 110:876, 1965
119. Koop CE: Observations on undescended testes. II. The technique of surgical management. Arch Surg 75:899, 1957
120. Rowe MI, Clatworthy HW: Incarcerated and strangulated hernias in children. Arch Surg 101:136, 1970
121. Koop CE: Inguinal herniorrhaphy in infants and children. Surg Clin North Am 37:1675, 1957
122. Snyder WH, Jr, Greaney EM: Inguinal hernias. In Mustard WT, Ravitch MM, Snyder WH, Jr, et al (eds): Pediatric Surgery. Chicago, Year Book, 1969, p 704
123. Mengel W, Hienz HA, Sippe WG, II, et al: Studies on cryptorchidism: a comparison of histological findings in the germative epithelium before and after the second year of life. J Pediatr Surg 9:445, 1974
124. Koop CE: Observations on undescended testes. I. Significance of the empty scrotum and indications for orchidopexy. Arch Surg 75:891, 1957

INDEX